Design For Inclusion

Volume 4

Series Editor

Giuseppe Di Bucchianico, Department of Engineering and Geology, D'Annunzio University of Chieti–Pescara, Pescara, Italy

The book series "Design for Inclusion" publishes studies aimed at untangling the complex relationships between design and society, especially with regard to human diversity and inclusion. The series cover the classical fields of industrial design, such as product design, interior design, service design and communication design, with a special focus on their interactions with other disciplines, such as the physical and social sciences. In particular, the series reports on the latest developments, both theoretical and practical, concerning different approaches to "Design for Inclusion": Universal Design, Inclusive Design, and Design for All. It shares insights into their multiple, interdisciplinary relationships with both the human sciences and the transversal frameworks and approaches typical of Human-Centered Design (HCD) and Design for Sustainability. "Design for Inclusion" addresses a very broad readership, including designers, engineers, architects, social scientists and stakeholders, who deal with any of the topics mentioned above and their various implications. It publishes volumes fostering scientific advances, as well as books devoted to supporting education and professional training. These include monographs, edited books and conference proceeding. Outstanding PhD theses on emerging topics, if properly reworked, may also be considered for publication. This book series is published with the support of EIDD - Design for All Europe.

Silvia Imbesi

Inclusive Design of a Smart Device for People with Parkinson's Disease

EIDD
DESIGN
FOR ALL
EUROPE

Springer

Silvia Imbesi
Dipartimento di Architettura
Università degli Studi di Ferrara
Ferrara, Italy

ISSN 2662-5644 ISSN 2662-5652 (electronic)
Design For Inclusion
ISBN 978-3-031-58251-6 ISBN 978-3-031-58249-3 (eBook)
https://doi.org/10.1007/978-3-031-58249-3

This Springer imprint is published by the registered company Springer Nature Switzerland AG
The registered company address is: Gewerbestrasse 11, 6330 Cham, Switzerland

Foreword

I've been working with Silvia Imbesi for many years. I met her when she was a student, and after her graduation she worked with me on several design research projects. She has always had a great sensitivity to Human-Centered topics and the field of design for healthcare and well-being purposes. After several significant academic experiences, she decided to participate in the doctoral program of the Department of Architecture of the University of Ferrara, in Italy, following the topic of Inclusive Design. As an Academic Professor in Product Design and as an expert in User-Centered Design for the Internet of Things, she asked me to be her thesis Supervisor, and I tried to accompany her on this stimulating journey providing my contribution to the planning of this complex project.

The research project she was able to develop is a fresh and novel example of the application of consolidated design methodologies to a complex, innovative, and inclusive design research project.

I created the acronym titling this work that I called PASSO (PArkinson Smart Sensory-cues for Older-users), in Italian meaning "step", referring even to the methodological and technological possibilities to take a step forward in the biomedical design research field.

The PASSO project aims to facilitate people with motor disabilities to train their gait and posture, thanks to an IoT system composed of smart devices sending sensory signals to the user and collecting data and information about the person's behaviors and performances.

After the doctoral program, Silvia Imbesi elaborated on the accomplished work and transformed it in this interesting book, precisely describing every single step of the complex design process, and providing a useful guideline for the development of a research project involving advanced technologies and peculiar human factors.

Giuseppe Mincolelli
Associate Professor
Department of Architecture
University of Ferrara
Italy

Preface

This book presents an applied research project aiming to promote novel inclusive approaches in the design of smart devices for healthcare purposes. Specifically, it describes the methodological User-Centered design strategies used for the development of the PASSO project, a multidisciplinary research project aiming to design multisensory cues and related smart devices for the gait and posture rehabilitation of aging people with Parkinson's disease.

The book retraces the project's methodological process, outlining and describing each step, from the planned objectives to the validation of the achieved results. This publication aims to be a useful case study for researchers tackling complex and multidisciplinary projects dedicated to fragile users, and needing a methodological sample on how to facilitate the interaction in a multidisciplinary team.

The project started during the author's doctoral research and is still ongoing. It presented novel results, encouraging the multidisciplinary team to continue the work, creating innovative design solutions in the field of mHealth systems using sensory feedback.

The institutions participating in the research project were the Department of Architecture of the University of Ferrara (Italy), the home institution of the Ph.D. IDAUP program, with the supervision of Prof. Giuseppe Mincolelli; the Department of Engineering of the University of Bologna (Italy), with the refereeing of Prof. Lorenzo Chiari; and ISNB Istituto di Scienze Neurologiche di Bologna (Italy), with the participation of Dr. Giovanna Lopane. The project took advantage even of the participation of other researchers, in particular, a big effort was put in by Mattia Corzani from the Engineering Department of Bologna, and his colleagues.

The design project related to the doctoral research regards an mHealth system called PASSO (PArkinson Smart Sensory-cues for Older-users), an innovative biofeedback system specially designed to rehabilitate gait and postural disturbances in persons with Parkinson's Disease. The system's target is PD subjects facing the initial and intermediate stages of the disease, dealing with several ailments but most of all with a physical decline that affects walking and general motor skills, impacting functional independence, well-being, and health-related quality of life.

The PASSO project follows an iterative User-Centered Design methodology: the design process of the project was split into three cycles, each one organized into four phases: planning (P1), analyzing (P2), creating (P3), and verifying (P4).

- Cycle 1 (C1): Sensory cues and system.
- Cycle 2 (C2): Devices submitting sensory cues.
- Cycle 3 (C3): System interface.

The involvement of users in the design process aims to improve the system's usability, allowing them to take advantage of a satisfying experience that will help them face, in a better way, specific activities of their lives.

The book's sections are dedicated to the initial purposes of the research project, its objectives, considerations about User-Centered Design methodologies, and the use of smart technologies for elderly people. Then, the three design iterative cycles are punctually described to help the reader understand the applied methodological process. Final considerations resume the most interesting aspect of this design experience.

Ferrara, Italy Silvia Imbesi

Contents

About the Author

Silvia Imbesi has gained a Master's Degree in Architecture, and a Bachelor's Degree in Industrial Design in 2008 and 2012, respectively, from the University of Ferrara, Italy, and a Ph.D. in Inclusive Design from the Department of Architecture of the same university, in 2023. Since 2009, Silvia Imbesi has worked as a freelance architect and designer, collaborating with other professionals, companies, industries, and institutions to develop projects and design research. Starting in 2012 to date, she has been working with the University of Ferrara as a temporary professor. In her role of research fellow at this university, she participated in many academic research projects related to Human and User-Centered methodologies, Inclusive Design of IoT-based Devices and Smart mHealth Systems, Design for the Elderly, and Design for Health and Wellbeing, among others. She attended a few international conferences as an invited speaker, and is the author and editor of more than 40 international scientific publications about innovative care solutions for fragile users and special populations.

1 Context and Methods

Abstract

This first chapter of this book describes the current social and technological perspectives on the design of smart devices addressed to elder people. Moreover, it considers several methodological approaches such as Human-Centered Design, User-Centered Design, and Inclusive Design, to provide a framework of suitable methods for this applied design research. The chapter also describes the concepts of usability, human factors, and user experience, as factors influencing strategies to put fragile users at the center of the design process. Finally, the author analyzes the Quality Function Deployment tool, allowing a comparison between qualitative and quantitative information, to establish which are the project's priorities, and which design factors can mostly influence its success.

1.1 Research Focus

This design research project focuses on the analysis and implementation of User-Centered methodologies to design smart solutions for older people. The research investigates how to increase the service's response to user needs, and how to improve the effectiveness of Inclusive Design for the elderly affected by Parkinson's Disease (PD).

The focus will be on the design of smart objects to help the elderly in empowering autonomy in daily life environments. Moreover, the author tries to identify and analyze the most suitable product types for the transition to the Internet of Things, as a bridge for the use of new technologies, combining the familiarity of widely distributed product types with innovation brought by new technologies today hardly usable by people starting to face a cognitive decline.

Specifically, the research investigates how to design a mHealth system for training and rehabilitating the gait and posture of people affected by PD, trying to preserve autonomy and postpone the need for personal assistance.

Objectives and Limitations

At the beginning of the research project, several main objectives were set to guide the design process:

(1) The definition of a User-Centered methodological process suitable for designers facing research projects related to aging users affected by PD, and also usable by multidisciplinary research groups carrying out research projects in the Design Research field addressed to niche users with specific requirements;

S. Imbesi, *Inclusive Design of a Smart Device for People with Parkinson's Disease*, Design For Inclusion 4, https://doi.org/10.1007/978-3-031-58249-3_1

(2) The definition of a design process considering the needs and requirements of older people affected by Parkinson's Disease, which can set guidelines for the design of non-medical devices for the improvement and short and long-term monitoring of the person's movement;
(3) The development of graphic strategies to represent obtained results during the ongoing project, testifying the process stages and improving communication between members of a multidisciplinary research team;
(4) The design, prototyping, and brief experimentation of a wearable smart device following the developed methodology with real users, as finalization and case study of the developed methodological process;
(5) The development of a non-medical device to be used primarily in non-medical environments because of difficulties related to the regulatory, health, and hygiene regulations, and due to the fundamental role that would have the medical competence.

Proposed Methodology and Expected Results

The User-Centered approach allows designers to directly involve users in every single phase of the design development, generating an iterative process where the user gives inputs that the designer translates into requirements and guidelines of the project. This process's outputs are tested and commented on by the user again (Norman and Draper 1986).

The User-Centered methodology was applied in this project, and its design process was divided into several phases. The first step was a planning phase selecting users and stakeholders and studying the context; then there was the analysis of users to obtain human needs, and the analysis of suitable technologies to identify technical constraints; Then, the creating phase was developed, defining design and technological solutions for the realization of prototypes; finally, during the verifying phase, developed prototypes were tested and analyzed to improve designed solutions.

The necessity of managing different issues related to several fields of knowledge makes multidisciplinarity a significant peculiarity of this project.

The described research is supposed to have a significant impact because of the large number of countries involved in defining timely strategies for the aging society. This research project proposes a meaningful method for researchers applying User-Centered methodologies to design products and services for aging people presenting degenerative syndromes. The considered research field is challenging because it integrates multidisciplinary and heterogeneous knowledge; the definition of a tailored methodological process seems an effective strategy for the design tools in this sector. Besides, if results are appreciable and usable for users on a large scale, it will have a valuable impact on the healthcare system by reducing expenses related to personal assistance, care, and hospitalization; and on the welfare system in the light of the increasing necessity of dealing with the incoming charges for the constant growth of the average age of the world's population.

1.2 Research Context

The widespread consumer culture that always induces us to replace what does not work as we would like, to throw rather than cure, to overcome rather than understand, is pervasive in all issues of our current society.

An obsession of contemporary civilization, and not only, is to remove everything that does not work optimally and is not highly efficient; in particular, the idea that time leaves signs that change the way things and people appear to us seems to be unacceptable.

Winning the signs of time, canceling its effects and its implications, seem to have great importance today: people try to feel less at the mercy of time by intervening where they can clear its signs, through modification of their own body (cosmetic surgery), through the look of their appearance (clothing), and through all aspects that are not perceived as satisfying.

The conflict of today's society with time, perceived as a debilitating and impoverishing event for the person, needs to be overcome by accepting and mitigating the negative effects that this brings, enhancing the positive intrinsic aspects that characterize it.

Design for the Elderly

The category of people currently embodying these concepts is the elderly, who are associated with the concept of the passing of time and represent a typology of fragile users. The design discipline has accepted the challenge of putting design to serve these categories. In particular, in the social field, we are witnessing a constant increase in the appreciation of niche users' needs, once considered marginal to those of the rest of society, which today represent a market with remarkable growth and a great development margin.

The average age of the world's population is constantly increasing, making studies fundamental for the development of innovative tools, services, and strategies to ensure an increasingly prolonged and qualitative life for the entire elderly population. It is therefore of great importance to find solutions to support and prolong the self-sufficiency and independence of older people in their own homes while limiting the costs of forced hospitalization and not necessarily reducing their security and quality of life.

In 2015 World Health Organization published the World Report on Aging and Health, a report outlining the framework for promoting "healthy aging" for the global population (World Health Organization 2015); this highlights that we need cross-sectoral actions to establish policies and programs to increase socio-sanitary assistance for the elderly in the perspective of long-term care. Expenditures in this field will be a wise investment since there are no economic and welfare tools to date to face the progressive aging affecting the world population.

According to the World Health Organization, life expectancy in the world has increased by five years since the beginning of the century, and design has to face the needs of the growing population of the elderly. This issue does not only mean trying to create more well-done and prestigious models of wheelchairs or stairlifts, but also considering every age as a stage to live at the best of our possibilities by fighting isolation, depression, and sedentary life. Design can be an effective tool to help make active life longer and to delay the need for care and hospitalization by increasing the autonomy and independence of older people.

Smart Technologies

The world is changing very fast: people are discovering new needs, technologies are developing faster and faster, and innovation is opening new scenarios for designing new ways of living and managing people's well-being. That condition makes it necessary to question traditional design methodologies and to think of new perspectives for conceiving services, strategies, and processes besides products.

The emerging technologies related to the Internet of Things are expanding the horizon of possible solutions for sustaining and prolonging the autonomy of people in environments they are accustomed to; technologies seem mature enough to allow the design of smart objects and smart environments that can adapt themselves progressively and autonomously to the needs of the person to meet their needs (Dohr et al. 2010).

Design Research has accepted the challenge of designing smart objects related to the Internet of Things field, with relevant implications on how many of the traditional product types will change in the coming years.

Smart objects are a valuable resource to increase the ability of constant adaptability of daily life environments to the specific needs of people living there because they can detect people's habits and autonomously decide how to personalize effectively.

In particular, this consideration refers to the possibility of satisfying the needs of the most disadvantaged categories of users such as older people. Smart objects represent a concrete opportunity to use the technologies currently available for the elderly, to help them to extend their active and independent lives and postpone the need for personal assistance, due to the progressive decay of cognitive and physical functions.

1.3 Methodological Approaches

Design Research is supported by a large number of methodologies focusing on people who will take advantage of designed products, services, and processes. Some of these methodologies are analyzed to find elements useful to this specific project.

Human-Centered Design

Human-Centered Design (HCD) is a multi-stage design process focused on human factors engineering, usability engineering, and user experience optimization. The definition of HCD is given in the ISO standard Human Centered Design for Interactive Systems: ISO 9241–210: "Human-centred design is an approach to interactive systems development that aims to make systems usable and useful by focusing on the users, their needs and requirements, and by applying human factors/ergonomics, and usability knowledge and techniques. This approach enhances effectiveness and efficiency, improves human well-being, user satisfaction, accessibility, and sustainability; and counteracts possible adverse effects of use on human health, safety, and performance" (00–17:00 2010). The cited standard defines six characteristics of the Human Centered Design process:

- Adopting multidisciplinary skills and perspectives;
- Clear understanding of users, tasks, and environments;
- User-centered evaluation-driven design;
- Considering the overall consumer experience;
- Involving consumers in the design and production process;
- Iterative design process.

When following the HCD approach, the designer is required to analyze and develop solutions for existing problems and test and validate the designed devices, services, or systems, to achieve planned goals in the real world (Ponce 2021).

Even if the human factor is the main focus of HCD, the process should also consider social and technological factors that interact together as human activities.

The HCD process follows three main phases that can be iterative:

Research: Analyze the problem and the user to understand the context and clearly define the problem;

Prototype: Suggest design solutions to solve the problem, prototype them, and test them with real users;

Implement: Plan how to improve the project based on the collected feedback. HCD is supposed to be the process of creating things starting from general natural characteristics and peculiarities of human psychology and perception.

User-Centered Design

User-centered design (UCD) can be described as a more focused version of HCD considering firstly the target audience ("FAQ: Human-Centered vs User-Centered. 2021).

The UCD approach places the person, including his/her expectations, needs, and requirements at the center of the methodological design process, the user is no longer intended only as a final user, but more generally as a person who interacts with the product or service during one or more phases of its life cycle. Considering this perspective, the output of the process modifies: it will not consider solely final products or services, but the total experience that the user enjoys at each stage of the project's life cycle will be designed, from ideation to realization, use, and disposal (Koreshoff et al. 2013).

UCD is characterized by a multi-level problem-solving process allowing the research and development team to analyze the user and context, and predict how the user will interact with the final products (Fig. 1.1). It also allows for verification, and validation of the design process output, considering the user's behavior in usability and accessibility in the real world (Norman and Draper 1986).

The designer has to help the user have a sustainable relationship with the product; to have that result, the designer must answer questions related to the user's needs including the following:

- Who is the user? Does the design reflect the user's characteristics?
- What is the product's user experience?
- What are the user's goals for using this specific product or service?
- When and how does the user interact with the product design?

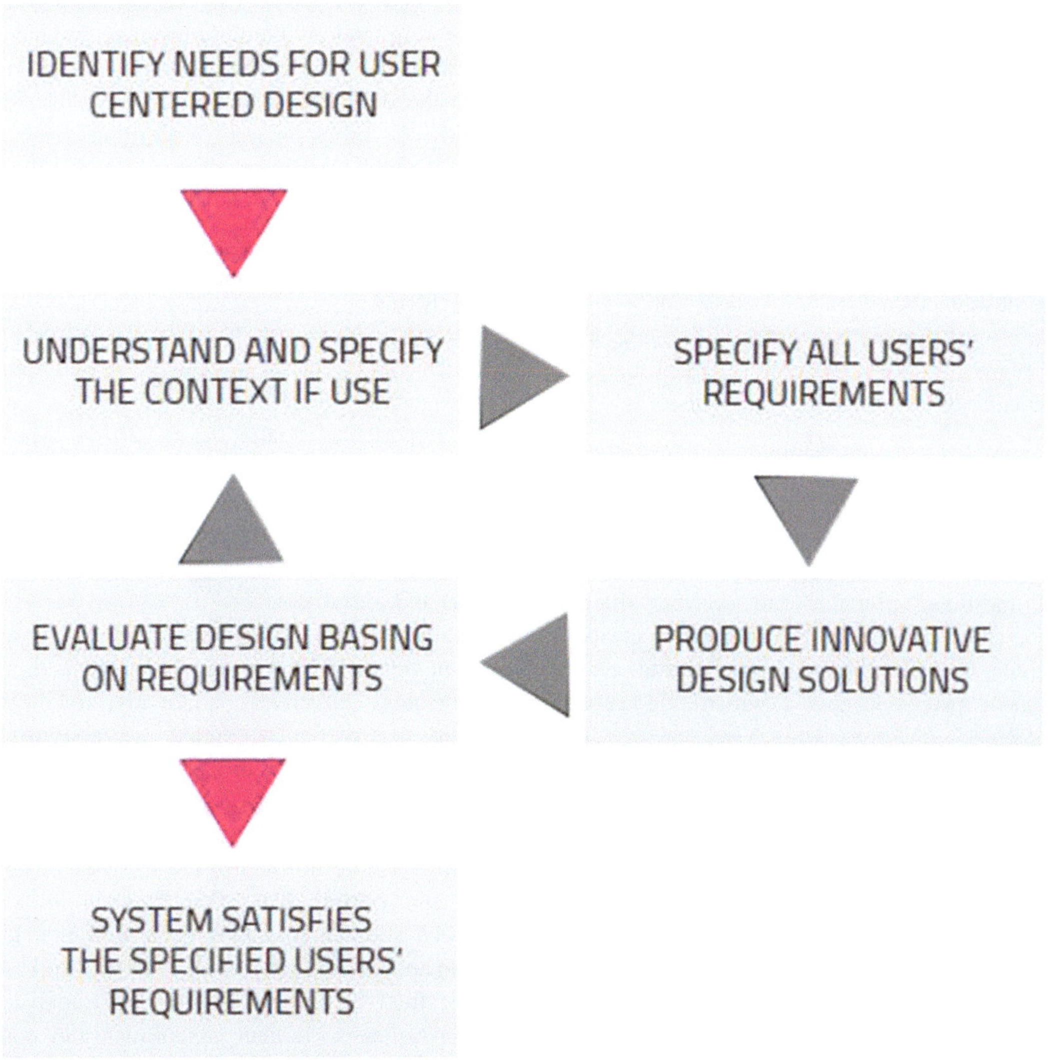

Fig. 1.1 User-centered design process

- How do the users think about the product or the design?
- Why should a person use this product or design?

The added value of UCD is that it facilitates individuals not requiring them to adapt their attitudes and behaviors to learn how to use the service, but the service itself is conceived to support and encourage the user to accomplish tasks, giving him a more efficient, satisfying and user-friendly experience (Goodman et al. 2007).

The design of devices, products, and systems in the healthcare field, requires a high knowledge of the capabilities and the necessities of the primary users; that information should be collected before and during the whole design process, to avoid design problems and reduce potential user's frustration related to the product ("Handbook of Usability Testing: How to Plan, Design, and Conduct Effective Tests, 2nd Edition | Wiley" 2021).

While HCD is based on involving within the design process all the people connected to the project in each stage of its life cycle, UCD is related to the involvement of the primary and secondary users in the design process.

Inclusive Design

Inclusive Design (ID) is defined as "the design of traditional products and services that are accessible and usable by the vast majority of people, without the need for special adaptations or specific designs" (Twitter and Facebook, 2005).

ID is a design and methodological approach very similar to that of Design for All (DFA), focusing its attention on increasing people's quality of life. This result is achieved by considering the needs and requirements of the end user from the very beginning of the design process.

The ID is used in Europe and considers not only disabled or elderly people, but embraces all those users having specific needs. Therefore, the greater the user's requirements, given by the different abilities/ disabilities of the users, the higher the relevance of the design method will be. It is common methodological practice, in the field of product design, to develop and design consumer products considering an average user; however, this excludes from the market a large percentage that does not fall within the classification of average users. ID, like DFA, instead seeks to place man, with his abilities, disabilities, tastes, needs, and needs, from the very beginning of the decision-making and design process.

In conclusion, "the principle of Inclusive Design, widespread in the United Kingdom, is close to the concept of Design for All but refers only to needs. It states that all environmental, engineering, and architecture projects, products, and processes must respond as much as possible to the diversity of human needs" ("Design for All. Il progetto per l'individuo reale - FrancoAngeli". 2021).

Usability, Human Factors, and User Experience

In UCD, it is important to consider three important concepts: Usability, Human Factors, and User Experience (Harte, et al. 2014). These concepts refer to how the user interacts with the product, service, or system, and how the design process should be ideated and developed to provide an experience that can give the user satisfaction and usefulness.

Usability refers to the extent to which a product can be used by the end-users "to achieve specific goals effectively, efficiently, and satisfactorily in a particular context. A usable product is easy to use, easy to learn how to use, and easy to remember how to use" (Harte, et al. 2014). The concept of usability was expressed for the first time in 1983 in the software design field, and starting from that moment its use has been adopted for many other design fields (Gould and Lewis Mar. 1985).

The field of Human Factors (HF) analyzes and investigates "human capabilities and constraints, investigating human features, structures and processes involved in interacting with

Table. 1.1: Scheme about Usability, Human Factors, and User Experience.

TERM	SOURCE OF DEFINITION	DEFINITION
USABILITY	International Organization for Standardization . ISO 9241S01: Guidance on Usability (1998) ISO; Geneva, Switzerland: 1998	"...the extent to which a user can use a product to achieve specific goals with effectiveness, efficiency and satisfaction....
HUMAN FACTORS	AAMI/American National Standard . ANSI/AAMI HE75:2009—Human Factors Engineering—Design of Medical Devices. AAMI; Arlington, VA, USA: 2010	"...the application of knowledge about human capabilities (physical, sensory, emotional, and intellectual) and limitations to the design and development of tools, devices, systems, environments, and organizations"
USER EXPERIENCE	International Organization for Standardization . ISO 9241S010:2010—Ergonomics of human-system interaction—Part 210: Human-Centred Design for Interactive Systems. ISO; Geneva, Switzerland: 2010	"...a persons' perceptions and responses that result from the use or anticipated use of a product, system or service" "...all aspects of the user's experience when interacting with the product, service, environment or facility"

designed artifacts and environments" (Harte, et al. 2014). HF can provide knowledge and models to empower design processes that aim to satisfy users' needs and requirements. HF involves other disciplines such as physiology, anatomy, cognition, and affective and social psychology.

The User Experience (UX) is the experience provided by using a device, service, or system. It includes the attitude to functionality related to the product usability, and also the affective and emotive dimension related to the product's ownership and use. "A positive User Experience provides the user with feelings of pride, value or self-efficacy while on the other hand, a negative User Experience can generate feelings of frustration, disability or stigmatization" (Harte, et al. 2014) (Table 1).

These concepts apply to the specific design context, always related but separated in their practical application (Fig. 1.2).

Quality Function Deployment

To integrate the UCD methodological approach, the Quality Function Deployment (QFD) was applied, which is used to allow simultaneous management of multiple users' needs and to translate intangible needs and qualitative requirements into concrete goals and measurable features (Akao et al. 1990).

The QFD is a tool that helps to design products and services starting from a hierarchy of users' and customers' needs (a customer is described as a person related to the product in one or more phases of its life cycle). The QFD allows feedback on the consistency of project proposals and starting objectives, both equally important aspects of this research.

QFD inputs are the "Needs", which are defined to reflect users' necessities, and the "Features", which are measurable performances of the object to be designed. Both needs and

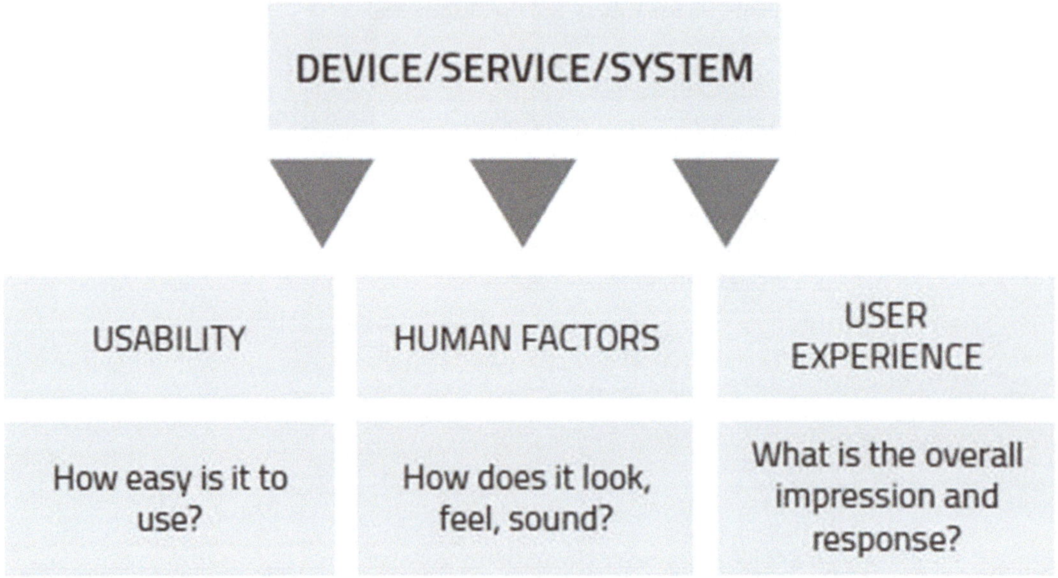

Fig. 1.2 Key questions in HCD design processes

features are put in correlation through a matrix chart, that helps designers evaluate the degree of relationship; starting from the hierarchy resulting from expressed evaluations, it will decide the performance due to items or services to be designed ("Quality Function Deployment - Franceschini Fiorenzo | Libro Il Sole 24 Ore Management 03, 2003—HOEPLI.it", www.hoepli.it. 2021). It is a visual decision-making procedure that enables a unique assessment of the user requests and a common consensus on the final technical specifications of the product. The use of this technique prevents long decision-making processes and costly project revisions and has the great advantage of being able to combine qualitative and quantitative data (Matook and Indulska Apr. 2009).

The general idea of this matrix was to make the needs expressed by marketing, design, and production coexist; where the expressed needs were present in the rows and the solutions to satisfy them in the columns.

The user (customer) is not only the person who will use the final product, but also the one who will produce it, assemble it, and advertise it. The user is "the set of all people who, at any level and any stage of its life cycle, have a relationship with the final product" ("Design Accessibile". 2021). To understand which are the main users of a product, it is necessary to carry out an analysis of the scenario and to know who will relate to the product throughout its life phase. This step should not be taken for granted, because finding and discovering users that other competitors have never considered can lead to the design of innovative products on the market based on unexplored needs. Once the users have been identified, a detailed description of each of them is carried out. This procedure, which at first glance seems obvious and banal, can innovate the quality of the final product: only by knowing the customers very well will you find precise, innovative, and fitting needs.

Needs and Characteristics

Once the detailed description of the user has been made, it is possible to proceed with the study of the needs, requirements, and expectations that the selected user has toward the product to be designed. This exercise is called "needs analysis" and aims to translate the information received from the user study into short sentences.

It is possible to identify three classes of needs:

Implicit needs: are those needs that the person tends not to think about when evaluating the product, as they are taken for granted. A failure to satisfy these needs would invalidate the whole value of perceived quality;

Explicit needs: These are the needs of which the user is aware, they are usually received through market surveys and direct interviews. These needs weigh heavily in purchase evaluations and constitute the predominant pattern of perceived quality;

Latent needs: These are the needs the person has, but does not know to have; the user is not aware of it just because there is still nothing on the market helping him to satisfy them. The identification of a significant latent need increases the perceived quality and can determine by itself an absolute competitive advantage.

There are several techniques for identifying needs. The choice of the suitable method for the final definition of the project output is a significant design choice since it is precisely from this analysis that the needs will arise, and then be translated into project human requirements, technical constraints, and specifications for the final creation of the product.

If there is the possibility of directly talking with the user, the personal interview is the most used technique as it provides a high number of requirements and maybe some latent needs bringing a high possibility of innovation. It is also possible to manage the interview with some users grouped into small families, to have a continuous comparison between the interviewees.

Regarding product analysis techniques, the users are questioned about how they use a particular product. Moreover, observing how products and services have been designed can help to understand innovative characteristics or weaknesses.

Every obtained need must be evaluated giving it a mark for its influence on the decision-making criteria for the realization of the final product or service. This phase is very delicate since entrusting a value to a need means classifying it as important and vice versa. The mistake not to make is to reserve a low score for apparently low need, which however could bring innovation to the final product.

Once all the needs that emerged from main users have been found and assessed, there is the phase of elimination of the needs with a negligible score, to reach about 20–30 total needs. A greater number of needs could cause severe organizational discomfort in the later stages of the work.

At this point of the process, are selected some characteristics related to the project output, indicated as a limited number of "concepts capable of defining a specific product performance in quantitative and measurable terms". In simple terms, they are all those aspects in which it is possible to quantify a product with a unit of measurement. It is also good that the number of features found for the object you want to design is in a number that is consistent with that of needs.

Matrix of Correlation

Once the list of the most important needs and the list of characteristics has been completed, it is possible to fill the relationship matrix. This tool is conceived to express how "technical decisions affect the satisfaction of each of the customer's requests" ("Quality Function Deployment - Franceschini Fiorenzo | Libro Il Sole 24 Ore Management 03, 2003—HOEPLI.it", www.hoepli.it. 2021). Therefore, it is possible to create a matrix table where the needs are inserted in the rows and the characteristics in the columns.

The task of the interdisciplinary project team involved in the QFD development is to evaluate the intensity of the relationship between needs and characteristics, observing how that particular characteristic (measurable and tangible concept) can interface with the need (intangible and immaterial concept) (Mincolelli et al. 2020).

The matrix of correlation can also be used to observe which features or needs should be considered more to obtain a quality and innovative product. The overall structure is called the "House of Quality" and contains all the considerations expressed up to now, represented by the following elements (Fig. 1.3):

	characteristic 1	characteristic 2	characteristic 3	characteristic 4	characteristic 5	...
need 1	0	1	3	1	1	1
need 2	1	9	3	1	1	3
need 3	3	0	3	0	9	3
need 4	1	1	3	3	9	9
need 5	3	9	1	1	9	3
....	0	0	0	1	0	1

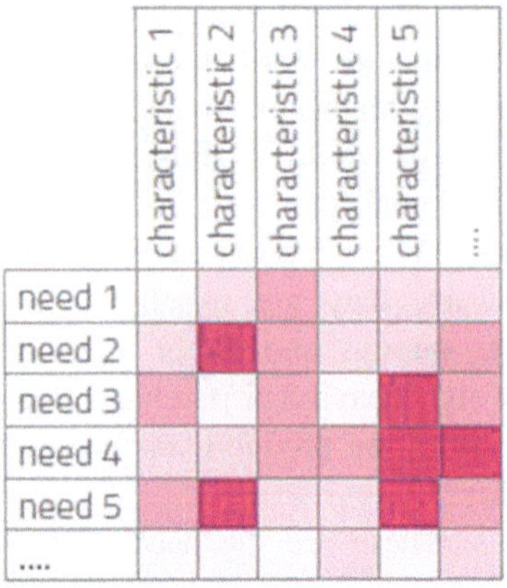

Fig. 1.3 Graphic representation of the QFD matrix using numbers or colors

Tree of needs (Customer Requirements): represents the needs analysis analyzed in the previous lines.

Needs assessment (Requirements Degree of Importance): Based on the methods listed above, the importance of each need is assessed. The values usually range from 1 to 5 (negligible; preferable; important; very important; essential).

Technical characteristics (Products Engineering/Design Requirements): The previously identified needs are translated into measurable and tangible characteristics.

Relationship Matrix: The relationship between each need and each characteristic is identified. The weight of the relationship is established using these values-symbols:

9 indicates a strong correlation;

3 indicates an average correlation;

1 indicates a weak correlation;

0 indicates an uncertain or absent correlation.

In conclusion, thanks to the Quality Function Deployment, we get to equip the team with a series of data and numbers usable to conceive innovative products and services without paying attention to any of the users who will interface with the final product.

Summarizing, this information is:

- a detailed description of the main users to whom the product is aimed;
- a list of all the needs, translated into technical specifications, of the main users organized hierarchically according to their importance (Customer Requirements);
- a list of product characteristics, organized hierarchically according to their importance (Product-Engineering / Design Requirements);
- the creation of the Relationship Matrix;
- a weighted analysis of the correlations between the characteristics (Correlation Matrix);
- A list of objectives in which the priorities of the project actions are analyzed.

1.4 Conclusions

This first chapter of the book analyzes design methodologies, such as Human-Centered Design, User-Centered Design, and Inclusive Design, that could be suitably applicable to this design research project addressed to niche users with peculiar needs.

The chapter also analyzes the QFD tool, which can be a really useful tool to match quantitative and qualitative information of complex multidisciplinary projects that need to consider many complex factors before the identification of the main project requirements.

References

D.A. Norman, S.W. Draper, *User Centered System Design; New Perspectives on Human-Computer Interaction* (L. Erlbaum Associates Inc., USA, 1986)

World Health Organization, *World report on ageing and health*. World Health Organization, 2015. Accessed: Nov. 27, 2021. [Online]. Available: https://apps.who.int/iris/handle/10665/186463

A. Dohr, R. Modre-Osprian, M. Drobics, D. Hayn, and G. Schreier, The Internet of Things for Ambient Assisted Living, *2010 Seventh Int. Conf. Inf. Technol. New Gener.* (2010)https://doi.org/10.1109/ITNG.2010.104

14:00–17:00, "ISO 9241-210:2010," ISO. Accessed: Nov. 27, 2021. [Online]. Available: https://www.iso.org/cms/render/live/en/sites/isoorg/contents/data/standard/05/20/52075.html

G. Ponce, "Field Guide to Human-Centered Design IDEOorg English", Accessed: Nov. 27, 2021. [Online]. Available: https://www.academia.edu/32807515/Field_Guide_to_Human_Centered_Design_IDEOorg_English

FAQ: Human-Centered vs User-Centered. Are the Terms Different? Tubik Blog: Articles About Design. Accessed: Nov. 27, 2021. [Online]. Available: https://blog.tubikstudio.com/faq-design-platform-human-centered-vs-user-centered-are-the-terms-different/

T. L. Koreshoff, T. W. Leong, and T. Robertson, Approaching a human-centred internet of things, in *Proceedings of the 25th Australian Computer-Human Interaction Conference: Augmentation, Application, Innovation, Collaboration*, in OzCHI '13. New York, NY, USA: Association for Computing Machinery, Nov. 2013, pp. 363–366. https://doi.org/10.1145/2541016.2541093.

J. Goodman, P. Langdon, and P. J. Clarkson, Formats for user data in inclusive design, in *Proceedings of the 4th international conference on Universal access in human computer interaction: coping with diversity*, in UAHCI'07. Berlin, Heidelberg: Springer-Verlag, Jul. 2007, pp. 117–126

Handbook of Usability Testing: How to Plan, Design, and Conduct Effective Tests, 2nd Edition | Wiley, Wiley.com. Accessed: Nov. 27, 2021. [Online]. Available: https://www.wiley.com/en-us/Handbook+of+Usability+Testing%3A+How+to+Plan%2C+Design%2C+and+Conduct+Effective+Tests%2C+2nd+Edition-p-9780470185483

Twitter, LinkedIn, and Facebook, *BS 7000-6:2005 Design management systems. Managing inclusive design. Guide*, Design Council. Accessed: Nov. 28, 2021. [Online]. Available: https://www.designcouncil.org.uk/bs-7000-62005-design-management-systems-managing-inclusive-design-guide

Design for All. Il progetto per l'individuo reale—FrancoAngeli. Accessed: Nov. 28, 2021. [Online]. Available: https://www.francoangeli.it/Ricerca/scheda_libro.aspx?Id=15809

R. P. Harte *et al.*, *Human Centred Design Considerations for Connected Health Devices for the Older Adult, J. Pers. Med.* **4**(2), 2 (2014). https://doi.org/10.3390/jpm4020245

J.D. Gould, C. Lewis, Designing for usability: key principles and what designers think. Commun. ACM **28**(3), 300–311 (1985). https://doi.org/10.1145/3166.3170

Y. Akao, G. H. Mazur, and B. King, *Quality function deployment: integrating customer requirements into product design* (1990)

Quality Function Deployment—Franceschini Fiorenzo|Libro Il Sole 24 Ore Management 03/2003—HOEPLI.it, www.hoepli.it. Accessed: Nov. 27, 2021. [Online]. Available: https://www.hoepli.it/libro/quality-function-deployment/9788883634550.html

S. Matook, M. Indulska, Improving the quality of process reference models: A quality function deployment-based approach. Decis. Support. Syst. **47**(1), 60–71 (Apr.2009). https://doi.org/10.1016/j.dss.2008.12.006

Design Accessibile. Accessed: Nov. 27, 2021. [Online]. Available: https://www.maggiolieditore.it/design-accessibile.html

G. Mincolelli, G. A. Giacobone, M. Marchi, and S. Imbesi, New Collaborative Version of the Quality Function Deployment: Practical Application to the HABITAT Project, in *Intelligent Human Systems Integration 2020*, T. Ahram, W. Karwowski, A. Vergnano, F. Leali, and R. Taiar, Eds., in Advances in Intelligent Systems and Computing. (Cham: Springer International Publishing, 2020), pp. 823–828. https://doi.org/10.1007/978-3-030-39512-4_125

2 Designing for Aging People with Parkinson's Disease

Abstract

In this chapter, the author describes impairments brought by aging and Parkinson's disease to older users, to understand how these impact the individual's senses, and to define the characteristics and requirements of this niche category of fragile users. The application of User-Centered Design methodologies to smart devices addressed to aging users requires a deep understanding of their abilities, and a correct analysis of their conditions to improve the usability of the product, service, or process that is going to be designed. The analysis presented in this chapter aims to define the aspects of motor and cognitive impairments that could be overcome by design and technological solutions improving the person's senses.

2.1 Considerations About Aging People

The research's case study has been identified in the project of a mHealth system for elder users affected by PD. Considering that one of the main PD symptoms is suffering from gait and balance problems, exercise is a valid help in improving gait and mobility in the short term.

To reduce the economic pressure on the public health system, given the increasing demand for services related to physiotherapy treatments, it would be desirable to have a smart device that could help the user practice exercises in their own house, to maintain, prolong, and improve the effects of the rehabilitation.

Following this perspective, it is fundamental to deeply understand and analyze the users' category of older people affected by PD.

Design for the elderly requires a high degree of usability, so the approach considered the most suitable for the development of this design and technological research project, is User-Centered Design (UCD), which helps design products and services in the most appropriate way for chosen users, characterized by peculiarities affecting the performance in using the objects most commonly used by the majority of the population (Mao et al. Mar. 2005).

Design Research has always had a deep connection with the detection and satisfaction of people's requirements, even if they belong to small niches of users characterized by specific peculiarities not diffused to the rest of the population. Within the Design Discipline, there are many possible approaches to empower the design process to gain a more effective response to users' needs and improve their quality of life, one of the most popular and experienced ones is Human-Centered Design (HCD), developed to be an approach on problem-solving that involves the human perspective in each stage of the design project (Ponce 2021). Citing the

S. Imbesi, *Inclusive Design of a Smart Device for People with Parkinson's Disease*, Design For Inclusion 4, https://doi.org/10.1007/978-3-031-58249-3_2

current standard, "Human-centered design is an approach to interactive systems development that aims to make systems usable and useful by focusing on the users, their needs and requirements, and by applying human factors/ergonomics, and usability knowledge and techniques. This approach enhances effectiveness and efficiency, improves human well-being, user satisfaction, accessibility, and sustainability; and counteracts possible adverse effects of use on human health, safety, and performance" (2010). Transposing this concept to the field of design for the elderly, HCD allows for the development of design processes that consider the affections of the older person's performances as invariants of this research project, not delivering this responsibility to the final user.

Global Ageing

Currently, the average age of people all over the world is constantly growing, bringing an increase in the demand for personal assistance and health care services for older people (World Health Organization 2015). It has never happened before that the average life expectancy was over sixty years (U. D. of E. and S. Affairs 2007), this is caused by the declining mortality among the elderly, in particular in the most developed countries (Christensen et al. 2009). This tendency is leading the whole society to significant consequences. Considering that changes brought by the demographic transition to the old population are predictable, it would be desirable to plan how to manage these social shifts positively and proactively (Beard et al. 2016). The aging trend requires a holistic public welfare answer: the scarcity of inclusive regulations and tools requires innovation to consent to a fair old age for all populations, without bringing an excessive burden on countries' public resources (Lloyd-Sherlock et al. 2012).

Some of the most significant aspects of the described trend needing to be rebalanced are the level of institutional costs and the quality of life of elder people. These objectives could be achievable by improving aging people's autonomy, helping them to live in their usual environment as long as possible, and postponing their necessity for personal assistance and hospitalization (Figs. 2.1 and 2.2) (World Health Organization 2015; Failed 2020).

Characteristics of Older Users

The current evolution of e-health and telemedicine is connected with the wide distribution of health-related devices and services addressed to the growing population of aging users for home use, prolonging their stay in their environment, and improving their quality of life (Harte, et al. 2014).

The definition of the main peculiarities and diffused habits of this category is fundamental to answer effectively their needs and requirements, using methodologies, approaches, and design tools developed and improved by Design Research.

The concept of aging refers to the biological, psychological, and sociological transformations happening in every person with the advance in chronological age. These changes usually affect the ability to detect, interpret, and respond to visual and auditory information, compromising the ability to carry out daily activities moderately or intensely ("Social Gerontology: A Multidisciplinary Perspective 2021).

It is quite difficult to find the values or characteristics that are exhaustive to define a person as an "older user": the chronological age is not a sufficient evaluation parameter, given the large range of changes in performances that could affect individuals, it is usually considered as an indicator of the modification of the social role of the person (Fisk et al. 2014). In most developed countries, the beginning of old age is roughly associated with the time of retirement, estimated at around 65 years. Nowadays this idea is slowly changing, starting to associate the beginning of old age with the point when an active contribution is no longer possible (Barrientos et al. 2003).

Designing for older people requires a big effort in analyzing their needs and requirements,

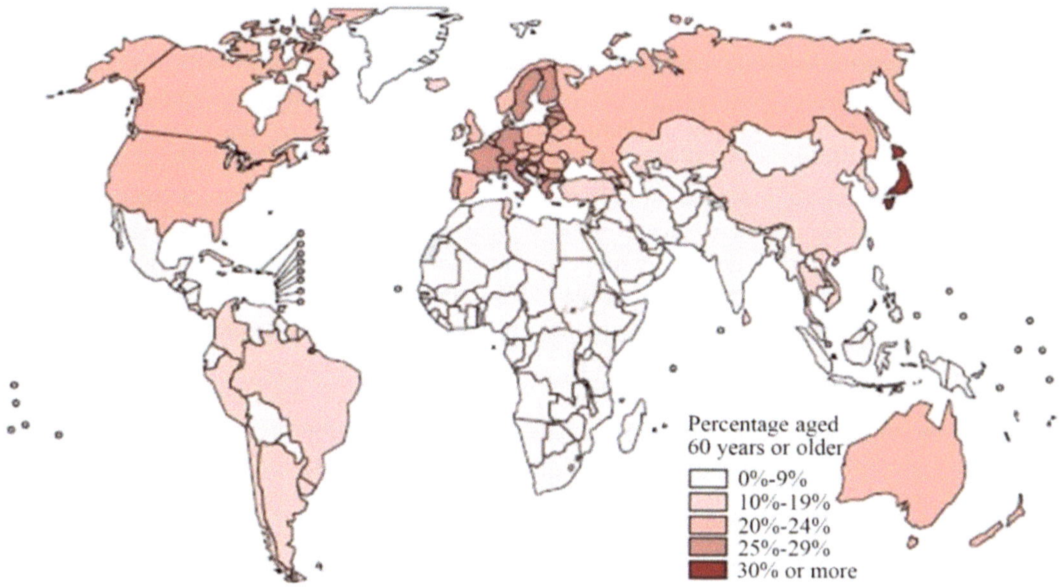

Fig. 2.1 Proportion of population aged 60 years or older, by country, in 2015. This image has been elaborated by the World Health Organization for the World Report on Aging and Health (World Health Organization 2015)

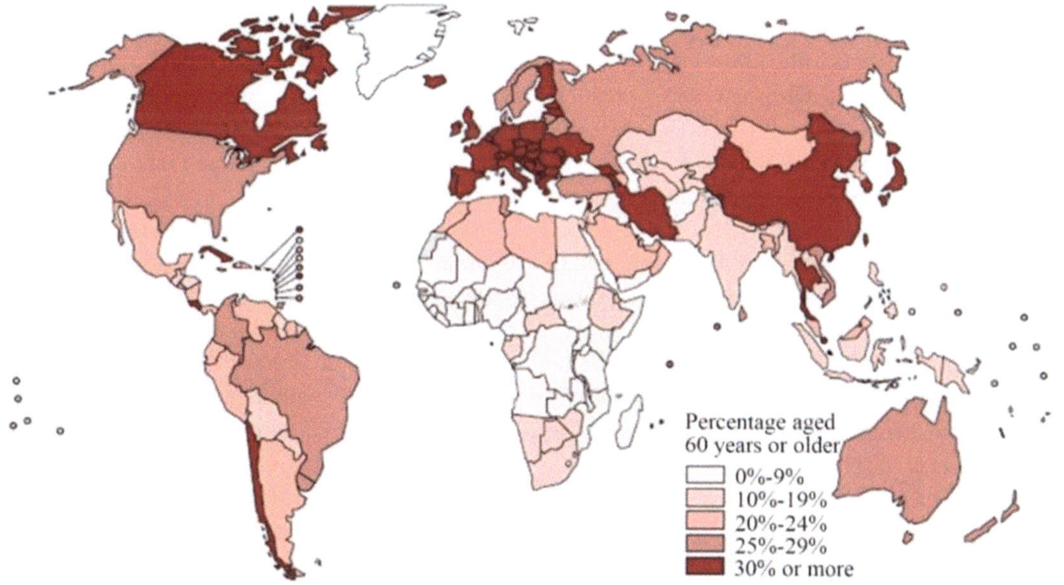

Fig. 2.2 Proportion of population aged 60 years or older, by country, 2050 projections. This image has been elaborated by the World Health Organization for the World Report on Aging and Health (World Health Organization 2015)

also in the light of the individual health status, that is why it is necessary to extend the study of the category at several levels including different knowledge fields (Hawthorn 2007).

The category of older people is various, including adults with different limitations in daily activities, but mostly independent in managing their tasks. There are many factors influencing the reasons why they decide to adopt a specific technological device, often not related to its real usefulness or its evident benefits to the healthy aging of the user (Thielke et al. 2012). It is therefore important to reflect on why some elderly refuse to use the most advanced current technologies, and why sometimes they do not take advantage of the healthier option when available.

Design Research has a significant role in developing solutions to help those people, born and grown with mechanical and electro-mechanical equipment, to improve their ability to interface with digital devices related to the Internet of Things (Sackmann and Winkler 2013).

When facing the use of smart devices, older users need to be open to an improvement of their digital skills; learning this kind of information, experimenting with new ways of interacting with products, and accepting different habits, are critical points influenced by the level of satisfaction in use that is linked to the user capabilities. The users' skills change across chronological age in terms of their perceptual, cognitive, and psychomotor capabilities. Those modifications influence the ability to interact with smart objects because they affect some senses like vision, hearing, and touch which are usually fundamental for an effective interaction (Charness et al. 2011).

Capabilities of Older Users

The capabilities of the user having the biggest impact on the level of interaction with a smart object are firstly the perceptual ones, and then, considering individual differences, psychomotor and cognitive capabilities. The main components of devices are software and hardware interfaces and instructional support, so the user needs to use vision, hearing, and touch to communicate with the product using its hardware interface, usually embodied by buttons, screens, lights, etc., to perform tasks. Depending on the level of success in the realization of the chosen task, there are two options: or the user's capabilities meet the task generating satisfaction, comfort, and a sense of safety empowering his will to continue the use of technology, or the smart device's demands exceed the user's capability, making him feel frustration, discomfort, and anxiety, resulting in the rejection of technology (Harte, et al. 2014).

Perception is related to the use of the five physical senses: sight, hearing, touch, smell, and taste. Sight, hearing, and touch are the senses involved in the interaction between the person and the elements that form his environment (Fig. 2.3).

Perceptual Capabilities

Sight

The largest part of the interaction with devices involves firstly the sense of sight, which with advancing age inevitably undergoes a decline, that is measurable as a degree of vision loss. To be more specific, several factors constitute functional vision and each one of them gets worse with aging.

Starting from the "normal" values of a person with an average level of performance, it is possible to estimate how the different components of sight deteriorate while the person ages and calculate the value representing the average factor by which the components will have generally deteriorated at a certain stage of aging (Brabyn et al. 2001). The most significant components to consider for the evaluation of sight deterioration are low contrast acuity (LCA), high contrast acuity (HCA), Low Contrast Acuity in Low Luminance (LCALL), Acuity in Glare (AG), Color Discrimination (CD) and Contrast Sensitivity (CS).

The modification of the personal sight condition implicates worsening changes in the effectiveness of the interaction with smart devices,

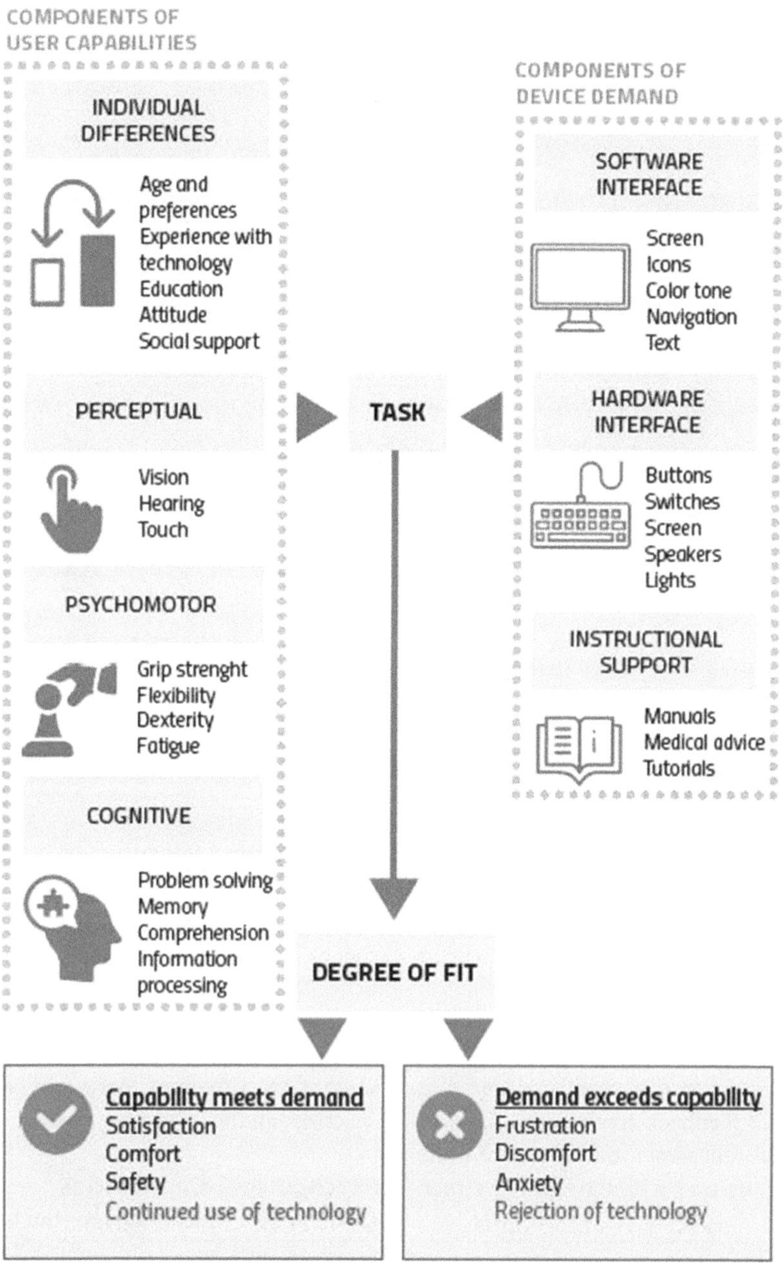

Fig. 2.3 User capabilities and device demands

in the following scheme are listed the main difficulties faced by the user in interacting with an interface (Fig. 2.4).

Hearing

There is wide documentation on the effects of aging on auditory function (Mitchell et al. 2011), documenting that hearing loss is very diffused, particularly in people over 75 years, and studying the relationship between the reduction of auditory function and cognitive decline (Tay et al. 2006).

The hearing level is usually measured by the evaluation of the personal hearing threshold, thanks to the measurement of the average

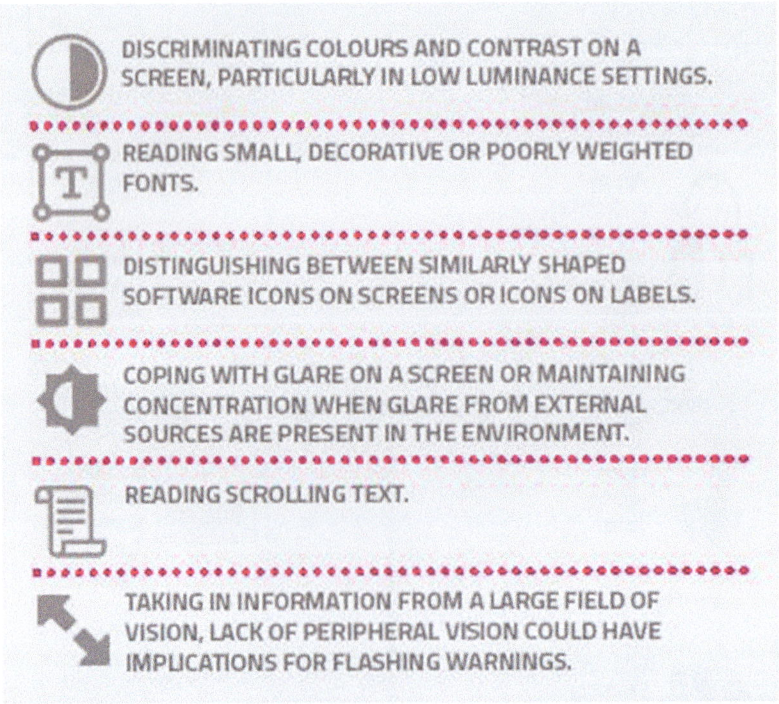

Fig. 2.4 Important issues related to sight in older users

minimum pure tone sound heard without background noise. That threshold increases while the person ages, reducing the values indicating the Decibel Hearing Level (dB HL) at a specific frequency (Kiely et al. 2012).

The changes in hearing performance affect the effectiveness of the interaction with smart devices that very often use sounds as an effective way to give feedback to the user. The following scheme represents the most common issues faced by the user with the hearing dimension (Fig. 2.5).

Touch

As the sense of hearing, the touch sensation is measured as the deviation from the threshold where an external stimulus is perceived by the users generating feedback from them (Wickremaratchi and Llewelyn 2006). In older users the light touch, vibration sense, and spatial acuity have an increased tactile threshold, causing a reduction in the touch sensation of the person (Kenshalo 1986).

Particularly, fingertips are affected by an impairment of the tactile threshold and a loss of spatial acuity, affecting the capability of the person to discriminate tactile details (Stevens and Cruz 1996).

The described decline has implications for the interaction between the user and smart devices, some of the situations that could cause issues are described in the following scheme (Fig. 2.6).

Psychomotor Capabilities

Psychomotor functions are fundamental when the user interacts with handheld devices, they are connected to the person's performances related to cognitive-based motor control, such as grip, dexterity, coordination, manipulation, and mobility of the upper limbs. The decline of psychomotor performance in the older user can be measured as a loss of muscle power, a decrease in the range of movement of the joints, and an increase in the variability of the finer motor movements caused by motor disorders (Harte, et al. 2014).

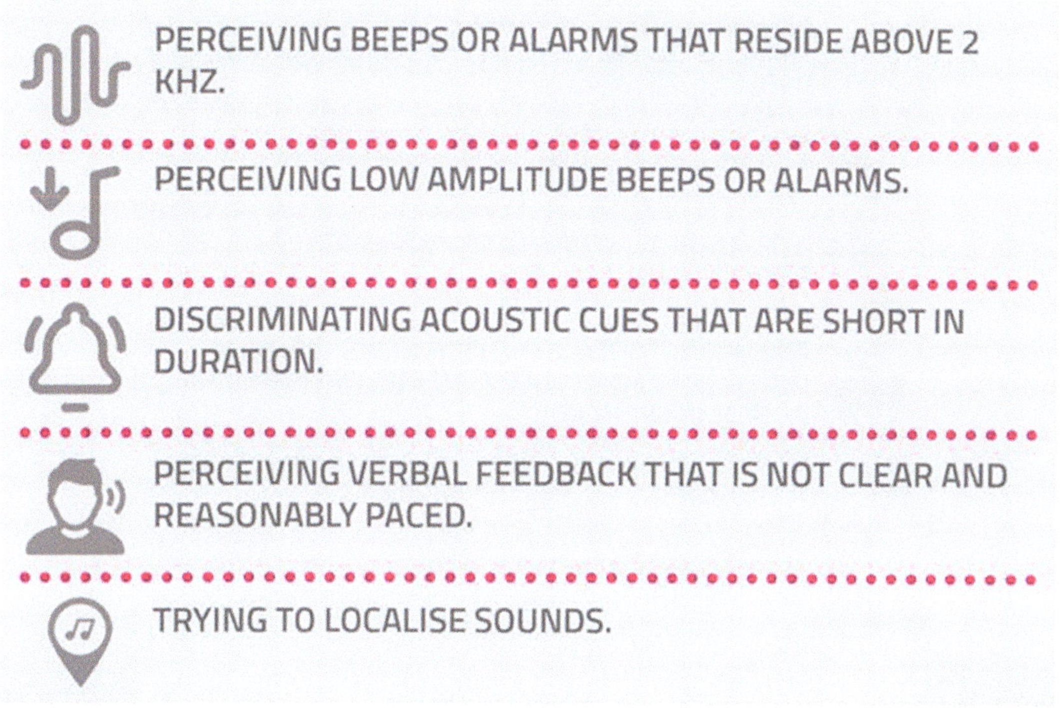

Fig. 2.5 Important issues related to hearing in older users

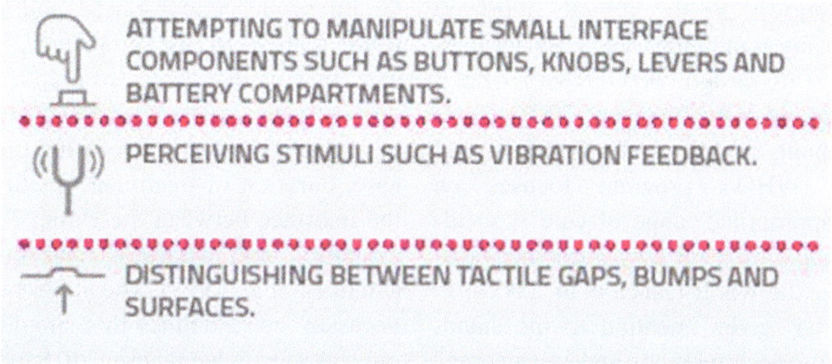

Fig. 2.6 Important issues related to touch in older users

The most essential actions on which the loss of psychomotor strength impacts are listed in the following scheme (Fig. 2.7).

The World Health Organization (WHO) is identified as an international and intergovernmental organization whose members are representatives of the United Nations, it was created in 1947 with the mission of ensuring everybody the best possible level of health, and of being an international authority for health matters, encouraging the technical cooperation between the WHO member states. The main responsibilities of WHO, as declared in its constitution, are: (i) to support governments in strengthening health services; (ii) to establish and maintain international epidemiological and statistical databases and services; (iii) to propose international health standards and conventions; (iv) to

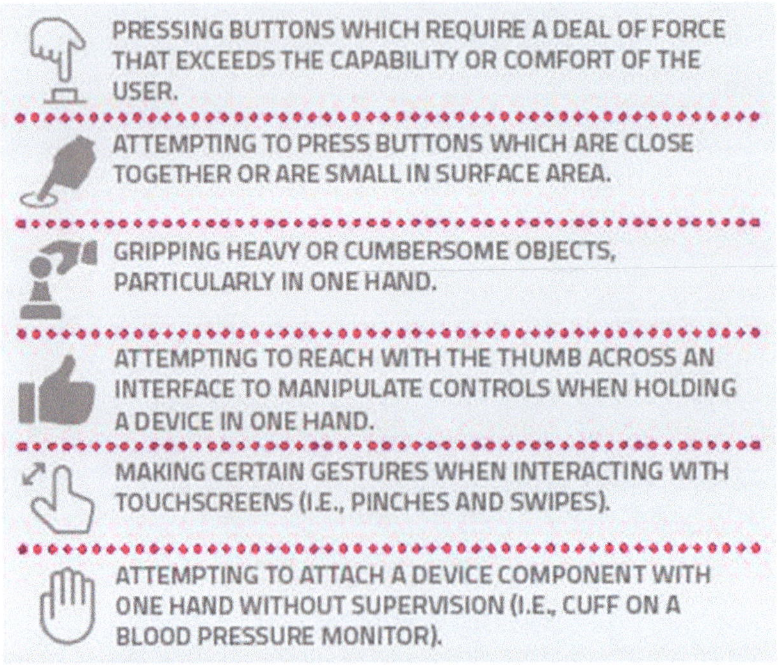

Fig. 2.7 Important issues related to psychomotor capabilities in older users

assist in the eradication of epidemic, endemic and other diseases; (v) to promote improved nutrition, housing, sanitation, and working conditions; and (vi) to design and conduct research projects in the field of health (Janca 2002).

Talking about neurological disorders and neuroscience, WHO's program focuses on ensuring an appropriate range of care is available to all people affected by neurological disorders all over the world (Janca et al. 2000), in particular, it has given attention to the standardization of research methods and instruments, and the development of guidelines and consensus statements on important research issues in the area of neurology and neuroscience (Janca 2002).

In the context of the Global Initiative on Neurology and Public Health, starting from 1997 WHO began to invest in activities related to PD. An important step was the creation of the WHO Working Group on PD including international experts, members of the European PD Association (EPDA), the World Federation of Neurology (WFN), patients with Parkinson's disease, and their caregivers. The Working Group produced consensus and recommendations related to the education, management, and costs of PD, they also emphasized the epidemiological research on PD that should focus on the relationship between the duration of disease, duration of treatment, quality of life, and the interface between the extent of impairment, disability, and handicap, and quality of life (Menken et al. 1997). They also highlighted the necessity of guidelines that should be based on our current understanding of factors and interventions, which have the greatest impact on the quality of life of people living with PD (Janca 1999). Similarly, without adequate knowledge of the burden represented by Parkinson's disease in the population as a whole, its treatment cannot be carried out in a planned way: traditional methods of prioritizing public health problems are usually based on mortality and prevalence rates and do not take into consideration of the non-fatal outcomes, severity, and duration of disability caused by the diseases. As a result, the public health importance of many mental and neurological disorders including Parkinson's disease has been underestimated (Janca 2002).

2.2 Considerations About People with PD

The users who will be considered in this research will be self-sufficient and non-self-sufficient elderly, their caregivers, and all the people who take part in their everyday lives, then will consider the needs of other people who have a less direct relationship with the aging person but are equally important, such as care center managers, healthcare operators, economic decision-makers, etc.

The first observation phase aimed to determine which categories of users the design of a smart non-medical device related to the Internet of Things would have the most appreciable impact. That device was conceived to help the older person autonomously carry out ordinary daily activities in his home environment, postponing his need for personal assistance and hospitalization.

Primary User: The first user will be the senior affected by PD, at the early stages of the disease, who lives alone or with a mate, but not with a person professionally taking care of him.

Secondary Users: Relatives of the senior (mate, sons, grandsons, and other people very close to the user); Healthcare operators and professionals as doctors who follow the person in a specific health field (neurologist, orthopedist, geriatrician, and other doctors taking care of the user), physiotherapists, nurses, and others.

Stakeholders: Public and private organizations caring about healthy aging, and promoting the diffusion of devices to be used in the early stages of the pathology.

Impairments of People with PD

When considering such a social and medical contest, it is important to deeply understand which physical factors can influence the relationship between the user with PD and other people and environments.

PD is a disease often associated with several motor impairments related to the gait such as akinesia (difficulty in starting the movement), bradykinesia (slow movement), rigidity, postural instabilities, tremors (rhythmic movements in a resting position), and events of freezing of gait (FOG) (Davie 2008). Together with these limitations, there is an increase in the falling risk and a general decrease in the quality of life of the person, starting to need personal assistance for activities of their daily routine (Campenhausen et al. 2005).

Motor Symptoms

As said before, PD users experience different symptoms but some of them, like bradykinesia, rest tremor, rigidity, and postural and gait impairments are usually present in all patients (Massano and Bhatia 2012).

Bradykinesia is described as a progressive slowness of movement speed, accompanied by amplitude while performing sequential and simultaneous tasks (Berardelli et al. 2001). This symptom impacts fine motor control abilities in everyday life, specifically on the ones regarding activities carried out with hands and fingers (J. J 2008).

Rest tremor is shown as an involuntary oscillating movement appearing when muscles are relaxed or supported. It usually doesn't regard fine motor capabilities and most of the time disappears when the action execution starts (Edwards et al. 2021).

Rigidity is increased resistance to the passive movement of a limb occurring during the movement and not related to its speed. Rigidity affects fine motor tasks and facial expressions and sometimes brings pain to the person (Association 2021).

Postural instability and gait impairment are common to the larger part of PD people, getting worse with the PD advances. The person tends to stand in a stopped posture, losing postural reflexes. The gait is slower and unbalanced while the stride length becomes shorter (Massano and Bhatia 2012). Another common symptom of gait impairment is FOG which happens usually in crowded or narrow spaces (Edwards et al. 2021).

Non-Motor Symptoms

Commonly, people with PD are shown to have sensory symptoms like olfactory dysfunction, pain, paraesthesia, akathisia, oral pain, and genital pain (Lee et al. 2006).

Even cognitive disorders are diffused in PD patients, leading to specific impairments starting from the early stages of the disease. The most common disorders are decreasing behavioral regulation in sorting or planning tasks, problematic use of memory stores, and defective manipulation of the representation of visual-spatial stimuli (Dubois and Pillon 1996).

Finally, dementia is described as a feature strongly associated with PD advanced stages and in aging patients (Levy et al. 2002).

On/Off Phenomenon

The on/off phenomenon is a relevant impairment related to PD, commonly appearing from the intermediate stages of the disease. The most common medication for PD is called Levodopa, whose effectiveness decreases over time due to lower absorption of the medication from the brain. The consequence is that the person switches from on phases, when Levodopa is acting correctly and avoiding symptoms, to off phases with a stop of the medication effectiveness and a consequent significant affection of the person's autonomy (Maziewski et al. 2009).

On/Off symptom oscillation	Contrast between On–Off phases
	Symptoms on Off
Disease progression effects	Autonomy loss
	Dementia
	Disease progression effects
	Multiple medication intakes
Possible consequences of PD motor symptoms on fine motor skills	Difficult repetitive movements
	Known problems using a mobile phone or other device with buttons
	Rest tremor
	Dyskinesia effects
	Rigidity and loss of dexterity
	Slow movements with fingers
Non-motor symptoms associated with PD	Apathy
	Attention loss
	Fatigue and depression
	Pain
	Planning problems
	Problems in vision
General characterization of a user with PD	Asymmetric symptoms
	Bradykinesia effects
	Different groups of PD affected persons
	Major symptoms
	Lack of balance problems

Fig. 2.8 Table reporting impairments and symptoms of persons with PD

PD Classification

The most common comprehensive tools providing a scale to monitor the PD-related degree of disability are Hoehn and Yahr scale (H&Y) and Unified Parkinson's Disease Rating Scale (UPDRS) (Walker et al. 2014). Then, for people's quality of life evaluation, there is the thirty-nine-item Parkinson's Disease Questionnaire (PDQ-39) (Ayena et al. 2017). To indicate the progression of motor abilities are generally used the Postural Instability and Gait Disorder subscore (PIGD) (Mancini et al. 2018) and Activities-specific Balance Confidence (ABC) scale (Nanhoe-Mahabier et al. 2012). Moreover, for the evaluation of cognitive decline are recommended the Montreal Cognitive Assessment (MoCA) (Mancini et al., 2018), the Mini-Mental State Examination (MMSE) scale (Rossi-Izquierdo et al. 2013), or the Frontal Assessment Battery (FAB) scale (High et al. 2018).

In addition to these kinds of classifications, more appropriate for a medical description of the patient, it is possible to classify people based on their impairments to get information on the ability to practice specific performances and to improve their independence in daily tasks. In a specific study, Nunes et al. analyzed users' performances and interviews to code results in a table showing all typical impairments of PD patients (Nunes et al. 2016). The creation of categories makes the impairments classification pragmatic, focusing on symptoms impacting daily life tasks, and allowing the design of devices facing those limitations (Fig. 2.8).

2.3 Conclusions

This second chapter describes the worldwide aging phenomenon, suggesting a growing attention to the specific field of design of smart solutions for elderly people.

Besides, it analyzes the most common impairments related to aging, especially referring to sense perceptions in relation to the use of smart devices and smart systems for healthcare purposes. Finally, it describes cognitive and motor impairments related to PD, to understand the characteristics and capabilities of this category of people, identified as primary users for the PASSO research project.

The design of a system using sense capabilities to rehabilitate the gait and posture of users affected by PD cannot ignore an eagerly awaited study on the possibilities of this category of users in interacting with digital tools to autonomously take advantage of a smart service.

References

J.-Y. Mao, K. Vredenburg, P.W. Smith, T. Carey, The state of user-centered design practice. Commun. ACM **48**(3), 105–109 (2005). https://doi.org/10.1145/1047671.1047677

G. Ponce, Field Guide to Human-Centered Design IDEOorg English, Accessed: 27, 2021. [Online]. Available: https://www.academia.edu/32807515/Field_Guide_to_Human_Centered_Design_IDEOorg_English

14:00–17:00, ISO 9241-210:2010, ISO. Accessed: 27, 2021. [Online]. Available: https://www.iso.org/cms/render/live/en/sites/isoorg/contents/data/standard/05/20/52075.html

World Health Organization, *World report on ageing and health*. World Health Organization (2015). Accessed: 27, 2021. [Online]. Available: https://apps.who.int/iris/handle/10665/186463

U. D. of E. and S. Affairs, *World economic and social survey*. UN (2007). Accessed: 27, 2021. [Online]. Available: https://digitallibrary.un.org/record/601358

K. Christensen, G. Doblhammer, R. Rau, J.W. Vaupel, Ageing populations: the challenges ahead. Lancet Lond. Engl. **374**(9696), 1196–1208 (2009). https://doi.org/10.1016/S0140-6736(09)61460-4

J.R. Beard et al., The World report on ageing and health: a policy framework for healthy ageing. Lancet Lond. Engl. **387**(10033), 2145–2154 (2016). https://doi.org/10.1016/S0140-6736(15)00516-4

P. Lloyd-Sherlock et al., Population ageing and health. Lancet Lond. Engl. **379**(9823), 1295–1296 (2012). https://doi.org/10.1016/S0140-6736(12)60519-4

S. Imbesi and G. Mincolelli, Monitoring Older People: An Overview of Devices Responding to Significant Needs of Elderly Affected by Parkinson's Disease, in *Advances in Additive Manufacturing, Modeling Systems and 3D Prototyping*, M. Di Nicolantonio, E. Rossi, and T. Alexander, Eds., in Advances in Intelligent Systems and Computing. Cham: Springer International Publishing (2020), pp. 646–656. https://doi.org/10.1007/978-3-030-20216-3_60

R. P. Harte *et al.*, Human Centred Design Considerations for Connected Health Devices for the Older Adult, *J. Pers. Med.*, 4(2), 2 (2014). https://doi.org/10.3390/jpm4020245

Social Gerontology: A Multidisciplinary Perspective, 9th edn. Accessed: 27, 2021. [Online]. Available: https://www.pearson.com/content/one-dot-com/one-dot-com/us/en/higher-education/program.html

D. Fisk, N. Charness, S. J. Czaja, W. A. Rogers, and J. Sharit, *Designing for Older Adults*. (London, CRC Press, 2014). https://doi.org/10.1201/9781482284775

A. Barrientos, M. Gorman, and A. Heslop, *Old Age Poverty in Developing Countries: Contributions and Dependence in Later Life*, (2003). https://doi.org/10.1016/S0305-750X(02)00211-5

D. Hawthorn, Interface design and engagement with older people. Behav. Inf. Technol. **26**(4), 333–341 (2007). https://doi.org/10.1080/01449290601176930

S. Thielke, M. Harniss, H. Thompson, S. Patel, G. Demiris, K. Johnson, Maslow's Hierarchy of Human Needs and the Adoption of Health-Related Technologies for Older Adults. Ageing Int. **37**(4), 470–488 (2012). https://doi.org/10.1007/s12126-011-9121-4

R. Sackmann and O. Winkler, "Technology generations revisited: The internet generation," 2013, https://doi.org/10.4017/GT.2013.11.4.002.00.

N. Charness, G. Demiris, E. Krupinski, Designing Telehealth for an Aging Population: A Human Factors Perspective. Boca Raton: CRC Press (2011). https://doi.org/10.1201/b11229

J. Brabyn, M. Schneck, G. Haegerstrom-Portnoy, L. Lott, The Smith-Kettlewell Institute (SKI) longitudinal study of vision function and its impact among the elderly: an overview. Optom. vis. Sci. off. Publ. Am. Acad. Optom. **78**(5), 264–269 (2001). https://doi.org/10.1097/00006324-200105000-00008

P. Mitchell et al., Five-year incidence and progression of hearing impairment in an older population. Ear Hear. **32**(2), 251–257 (2011). https://doi.org/10.1097/AUD.0b013e3181fc98bd

T. Tay, J.J. Wang, A. Kifley, R. Lindley, P. Newall, P. Mitchell, Sensory and cognitive association in older persons: findings from an older Australian population. Gerontology **52**(6), 386–394 (2006). https://doi.org/10.1159/000095129

K.M. Kiely, B. Gopinath, P. Mitchell, M. Luszcz, K.J. Anstey, Cognitive, health, and sociodemographic predictors of longitudinal decline in hearing acuity among older adults. J. Gerontol. A Biol. Sci. Med. Sci. **67**(9), 997–1003 (2012). https://doi.org/10.1093/gerona/gls066

M.M. Wickremaratchi, J.G. Llewelyn, Effects of ageing on touch. Postgrad. Med. J. **82**(967), 301–304 (2006). https://doi.org/10.1136/pgmj.2005.039651

D.R. Kenshalo, Somesthetic sensitivity in young and elderly humans. J. Gerontol. **41**(6), 732–742 (1986). https://doi.org/10.1093/geronj/41.6.732

J.C. Stevens, L.A. Cruz, Spatial acuity of touch: ubiquitous decline with aging revealed by repeated threshold testing. Somatosens. Mot. Res. **13**(1), 1–10 (1996). https://doi.org/10.3109/08990229609028907

A. Janca, Parkinson's disease from WHO perspective and a public health point of view. Parkinsonism Relat. Disord. **9**(1), 3–6 (2002). https://doi.org/10.1016/s1353-8020(02)00038-x

A. Janca, L. Prilipko, B. Saraceno, A World Health Organization perspective on neurology and neuroscience. Arch. Neurol. **57**(12), 1786–1788 (2000). https://doi.org/10.1001/archneur.57.12.1786

M. Menken, A. Janca, W. H. O. D. of M. Health, and S. WHO Working Group on Parkinson's Disease Meeting (1997 : Geneva, "Parkinson's disease and public health : educational and management implications," World Health Organization, WHO/MSA/MNH/NRS/97.6, 1997. Accessed: 27, 2021. [Online]. Available: https://apps.who.int/iris/handle/10665/63572

A. Janca, A report on the WHO working group on Parkinson's disease. Neuroepidemiology **18**(5), 236–240 (1999). https://doi.org/10.1159/000026217

C.A. Davie, A review of Parkinson's disease. Br. Med. Bull. **86**(1), 109–127 (2008). https://doi.org/10.1093/bmb/ldn013

S. von Campenhausen et al., Prevalence and incidence of Parkinson's disease in Europe. Eur. Neuropsychopharmacol. **15**(4), 473–490 (2005). https://doi.org/10.1016/j.euroneuro.2005.04.007

J. Massano, K.P. Bhatia, Clinical approach to Parkinson's disease: features, diagnosis, and principles of management. Cold Spring Harb. Perspect. Med. **2**(6), a008870 (2012). https://doi.org/10.1101/cshperspect.a008870

A. Berardelli, J.C. Rothwell, P.D. Thompson, M. Hallett, Pathophysiology of bradykinesia in Parkinson's disease. Brain J. Neurol. **124**(Pt), 2131–2146 (2001). https://doi.org/10.1093/brain/124.11.2131

J. J, Parkinson's disease: clinical features and diagnosis, *J. Neurol. Neurosurg. Psychiatry*, 79(4) (2008). https://doi.org/10.1136/jnnp.2007.131045

M. Edwards, N. Quinn, and K. Bhatia, *Parkinson's Disease and Other Movement Disorders (Oxford Specialist Handbooks in Neurology)*. Oxford University Press. Accessed: 26, 2021. [Online]. Available: https://oxfordmedicine.com/view/10.1093/med/9780198569848.001.0001/med-9780198569848

E. P. D. Association, *The European Parkinson's Disease Standards of Care Consensus Statement*. Accessed: 28, 2021. [Online]. Available: https://www.epda.eu.com/latest/resources/the-european-parkinsons-disease-standards-of-care-consensus-statement/

P.H. Lee, S.H. Yeo, H.J. Kim, H.Y. Youm, Correlation between cardiac 123I-MIBG and odor identification in patients with Parkinson's disease and multiple system atrophy. Mov. Disord. **21**(11), 1975–1977 (2006). https://doi.org/10.1002/mds.21083

B. Dubois, B. Pillon, Cognitive deficits in Parkinson's disease. J. Neurol. **244**(1), 2–8 (1996). https://doi.org/10.1007/PL00007725

G. Levy et al., Combined effect of age and severity on the risk of dementia in Parkinson's disease. Ann. Neurol. **51**(6), 722–729 (2002). https://doi.org/10.1002/ana.10219

P. Maziewski, P. Suchomski, B. Kostek, and A. Czyzewski, An intuitive graphical user interface for the Parkinson's Disease patients, in *2009 4th International IEEE/EMBS Conference on Neural Engineering*, (2009), pp. 14–17. https://doi.org/10.1109/NER.2009.5109223

R.W. Walker, R. Zietsma, W.K. Gray, Could a new sensory pen assist in the early diagnosis of Parkinson's? Expert Rev. Med. Devices **11**(3), 243–245 (2014). https://doi.org/10.1586/17434440.2014.900437

J.C. Ayena, L.E. Tremblay, M.J.-D. Otis, B.-A.J. Ménélas, Comparing auditory, visual and vibrotactile cues in individuals with Parkinson's disease for reducing risk of falling over different types of soil. Somatosens. Mot. Res. **34**(4), 226–234 (2017). https://doi.org/10.1080/08990220.2017.1421157

M. Mancini, K. Smulders, G. Harker, S. Stuart, J.G. Nutt, Assessment of the ability of open- and closed-loop cueing to improve turning and freezing in people with Parkinson's disease. Sci. Rep. **8**(1), 12773 (2018). https://doi.org/10.1038/s41598-018-31156-4

W. Nanhoe-Mahabier, J.H. Allum, E.P. Pasman, S. Overeem, B.R. Bloem, The effects of vibrotactile biofeedback training on trunk sway in Parkinson's disease patients. Parkinsonism Relat. Disord. **18**(9), 1017–1021 (2012). https://doi.org/10.1016/j.parkreldis.2012.05.018

M. Rossi-Izquierdo et al., Vibrotactile neurofeedback balance training in patients with Parkinson's disease: Reducing the number of falls. Gait Posture **37**(2), 195–200 (2013). https://doi.org/10.1016/j.gaitpost.2012.07.002

C.M. High, H.F. McHugh, S.C. Mills, S. Amano, J.E. Freund, S. Vallabhajosula, Vibrotactile Feedback Alters Dynamics Of Static Postural Control In Persons With Parkinson's Disease But Not Older Adults At High Fall Risk. Gait Posture **63**, 202–207 (2018). https://doi.org/10.1016/j.gaitpost.2018.05.010

F. Nunes, P. A. Silva, J. Cevada, A. Correia Barros, and L. Teixeira, User interface design guidelines for smartphone applications for people with Parkinson's disease, *Univers. Access Inf. Soc.*, 15(4), pp. 659–679 (2016). https://doi.org/10.1007/s10209-015-0440-1

3 Benchmark of Smart Devices for Parkinson's Disease

Abstract

Technologies for aging users require a high degree of usability, especially if considering smart solutions characterized by a high level of innovation and digitalization. In this chapter, the author analyzes several smart devices specifically conceived to improve the gait and posture of people affected by Parkinson's disease. The selected products are Personal KinetiGraph, Path Finder, Emma Watch, and Gyroglove. All considered smart devices were designed using a User-Centered methodology, involving users in parts of the design process. These products were selected as benchmarking of the research project, and selected as inspirations for the development of the PASSO project.

3.1 Technologies for Ageing Users

Currently, different instruments to monitor physical parameters are available as widespread products or innovative design concepts. These devices have several critical points, related to the design approach where mechanical and engineering aspects are considered as the main priority, at the expense of the empathic, functional, and aesthetic aspects. That is why many of these products still need to achieve the desired success.

With the development of smart objects and the Internet of Things (IoT), it is now possible to design devices interconnected with the network (Xu et al. 2014); designers who are willing to apply these new technologies will unavoidably have to think about new ways of engaging the user, new rules, and communication paradigms (Borsci and Federici 2008). At present, it seems to be indispensable to look for solutions that employ new technologies to satisfy users' needs and allow them to design products that can improve the quality of people's lives.

The studies and scientific research on cognitive ergonomics carried out in recent years confirm that the study of human/machine interaction is becoming increasingly important (Rizzo 1994). In addition, we are assisting the progressive transfer of healthcare and assistance issues from the medical context to the domestic one, and this is going to have relevant repercussions on how homes, furniture, and home devices addressed to the elderly are designed.

Current technologies have a central role in developing HCD solutions: their constant evolution creates continuous new possibilities for application and technology transfer. The concept of the Internet is evolving from "a network of interconnected computers to a network of interconnected objects" (Association 2021), giving birth to the Internet of Things, a platform including daily objects, devices, environments, and services (Imbesi and Scataglini 2021).

S. Imbesi, *Inclusive Design of a Smart Device for People with Parkinson's Disease*, Design For Inclusion 4, https://doi.org/10.1007/978-3-031-58249-3_3

A growing portion of the IoT is dedicated to consumer applications, especially regarding the Smart Home, making possible a connection between different devices to help the user improve his status of health and well-being. Referring to design for aging people, the IoT gives designers a huge amount of new possibilities in creating smart solutions for the daily monitoring of the person in the daily environment. The choice of an HCD approach in those typologies of design projects seems to be useful in the expansion of the effectiveness of the conceived design solutions and addresses specific users (Koreshoff et al. 2013).

The ongoing global aging has as a consequence the increasing need for home smart assistance, as the one offered by healthcare devices associated with specific pathologies, able to improve the person's autonomy and unburden the impact on the public healthcare system (World Health Organization, World report on ageing and health 2015). The recent developments in the e-health and telemedicine fields can facilitate the shift of several healthcare services from the medical context to the patient's home (Thomson et al. 2013), improving the efficiency of prevention and self-monitoring (Dorr et al. 2007), and transforming the care process into a continuous collaborative relationship between patients and healthcare providers (Charness et al. 2011).

The fundamental role of prevention in the graying society, suggests an improvement of Design Research both in the medical field and in the in-home self-care one: the growing importance of devices helping older people to prevent and manage diseases of chronic medical conditions, leads to new opportunities of innovation in the development of solutions for daily problems of niche categories of users. Scientific literature presents many studies on how significant can be innovative technology in motivating older people to adopt a healthier lifestyle, especially in conditions such as obesity, diabetes, etc., providing the user information elaborated from the collected data for the own management of healthcare conditions (Hurling et al. 2007; Imbesi and Mincolelli 2020).

3.2 Benchmark of Innovative Products for PD

Currently, there are still no tested and commercially available solutions for smart-based support and support systems that are completely able to assist the elderly by monitoring and interpreting behaviors based on measurable parameters, making choices through artificial intelligence, and providing assistance in a discreet, not intrusive or coercive way.

Active objects with natural interaction and a web-based remote resource system would allow older users a safe and autonomous stay in their usual habitation locations, promoting interaction with family and healthcare professionals. In particular, the goal of realizing and installing monitoring systems providing real-time assistive actions has not been widely achieved, except through purely functional, medical-hospital objects and systems (Pollini et al. 2022).

The objective of the benchmark analysis presented in this chapter is to evaluate some design solutions currently available in the market and to verify how they fit the requirements that have been identified (Mincolelli et al. 2018). The health-related smart devices state-of-the-art was analyzed, considering the ones used to help the elderly during their gait and monitoring their movements for short and long-term evaluations. The design process, the styling, the used technologies, the level of usability, the interface for the user, and the actual or potential diffusion on the market were analyzed.

The products chosen for comparison met the following criteria:

- There is a direct interaction between the person and the product;
- The product is usable autonomously by the older person;
- The product gives instantaneous feedback to the user on its usefulness;
- The product has the double function of facilitating the user in a specific daily activity and, on the other side, collecting data for a long-term movement analysis of the person.

Personal KinetiGraph

This wearable device is called the Personal KinetiGraph (PKG) (Fig. 3.1). It is a wrist-worn device recording data on the patient's movements in a maximum 10-day period (Emily 2023). It is conceived to provide a continuous ambulatory assessment of the treatable and disabling symptoms such as tremors, slow or involuntary movements, motor skills fluctuations, and immobility. The collected data regarding motor symptoms are elaborated and sent to the healthcare professionals assisting the patient. This solution allows for more informed treatment decisions, a potential improvement of the person's quality of life, and can reduce costs along the healthcare continuum.

The device has been tested and improved along several production phases, and the results of this experimentation are reported in three main studies: the study "Objective Data in Parkinson's Disease: A description of over 20,000 Parkinson's symptom scores across the World using the PKG", is the most extended one and shows updated results from that growing database, involving 21,234 PKG users worldwide for 6 years. The other two considered studies are "Costs and outcomes for Parkinson's disease patients who have their management adjusted by PKG" and "Pilot economic evaluation of PKG for management of Parkinson's disease in Australia". These publications describe this product as having the potential to provide clinicians with a passive and continuous assessment of patients' symptoms, helping them to better understand disease progression and optimize treatments, improving motor symptom management.

Publications also tried to assess the potential amount of cost savings with satisfying results, considering that even a small change in therapy provides a small benefit for the patient, and allows a reduction of annual therapy costs for the individual and for the whole healthcare system (Pahwa et al. 2018).

Path Finder

Path Finder is composed of two devices that should be attached to the user's shoes to help people affected by PD in the walk ("Path Finder|Innovative Walking Aid For Parkinson's Disease" 2023) (Fig. 3.2). One of the main

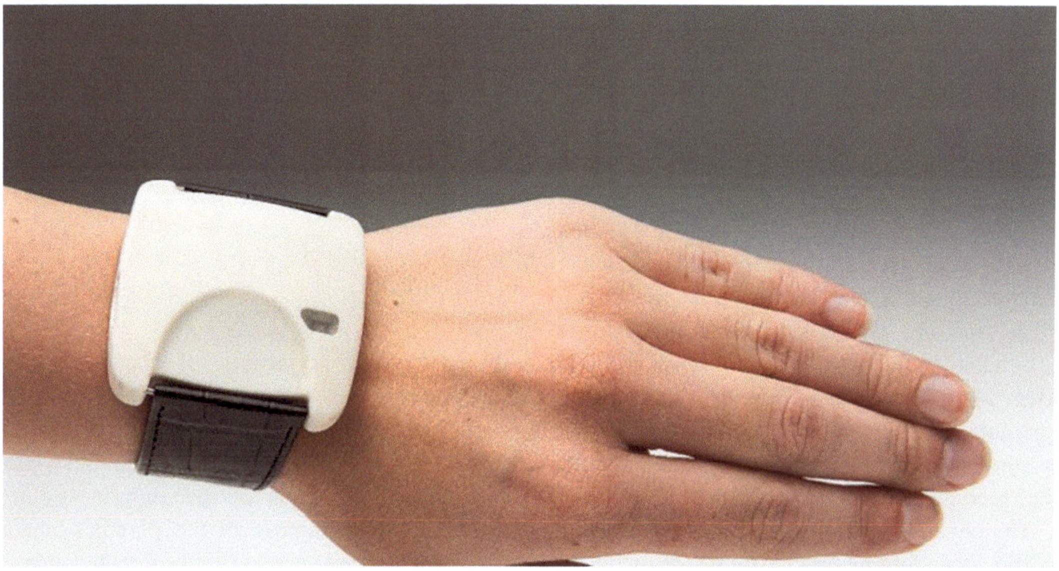

Fig. 3.1 The Personal KinetiGraph (PKG) has been produced by Global Kinetics since 2012. The prototype was developed by Grey Innovation and Florey Neuroscience Institute in Melbourne, Australia (Emily 2023)

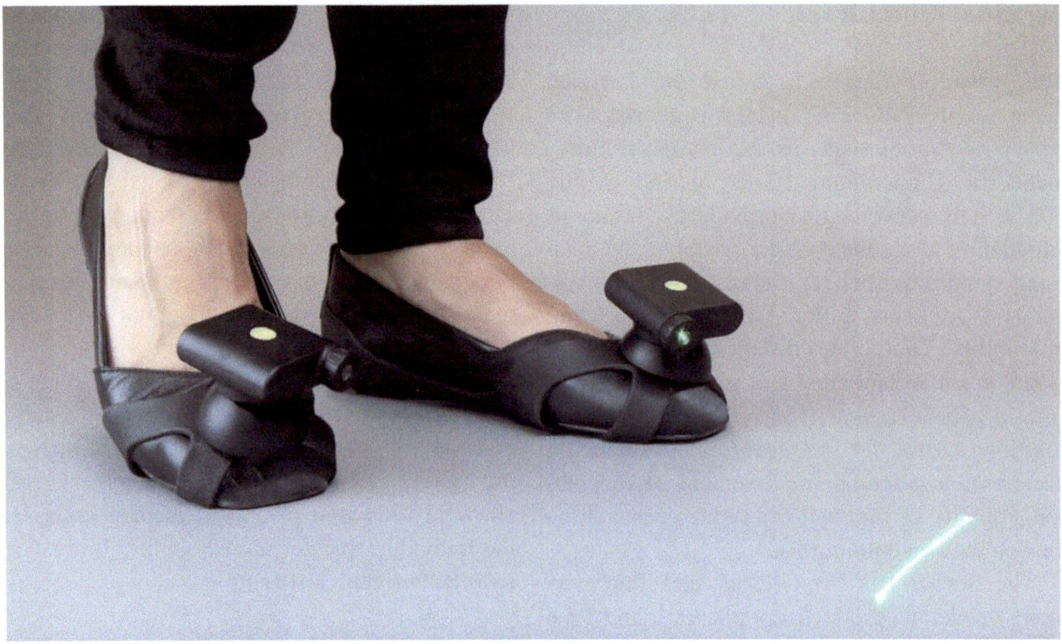

Fig. 3.2 Path Finder, a device that helps people with Parkinson's disease to overcome freezing of the gait. The first concept was designed by the graduating design student Lisa Pape ("Path Finder|Innovative Walking Aid For Parkinson's Disease" 2023)

symptoms of PD is the worsening of the gait, which assumes a typical walk aspect: this change is called freezing of gait (FoG) and results in the person appearing like he or she is stuck to the ground. Path Finder is a shoe attachment containing a laser that projects visual cues onto the floor to guide subsequent stepping movement of the adjacent leg. Its aim is the reduction of FoG and falling episodes in PD patients. The device is placed on a strap that is attached to each shoe. It works by projecting a green laser line in front of the opposing foot, providing a visual obstacle over which the user should aim to step. The device aims to trigger walking by focusing the attention of the user thanks to the provision of a visual cue. The lasers are activated by each step and provide continuous cueing while walking. Path Finder operates on a rechargeable battery and the company recommends users charge the unit daily.

The physical testing with users began to verify the concept of using visual cues to overcome Freezing of the Gait, using just black strips of tape placed in a walking pattern. The company describes marked improvements in several aspects: step length, overall gait stability, and regularity, evaluating the difference by observation. Another in-house study demonstrated the efficacy of Path Finder in decreasing the number of freezing episodes in a given obstacle course (Davis 2018).

Although Path Finder has only been tested with PD patients thus far, scientific literature suggests a potential benefit for a wider range of users with movement disorders.

Emma Watch

Another typical symptom of Parkinson's is the constant presence of shaking and tremors. To mitigate the impact of this disease, Haiyan Zhang designed a device called Emma, which has the name of the person inventing it, to compensate for the tremors in the person's hands (Fig. 3.3). Emma was initially created for a British graphic designer, whose Parkinson's disease had left her unable to do her job. Emma

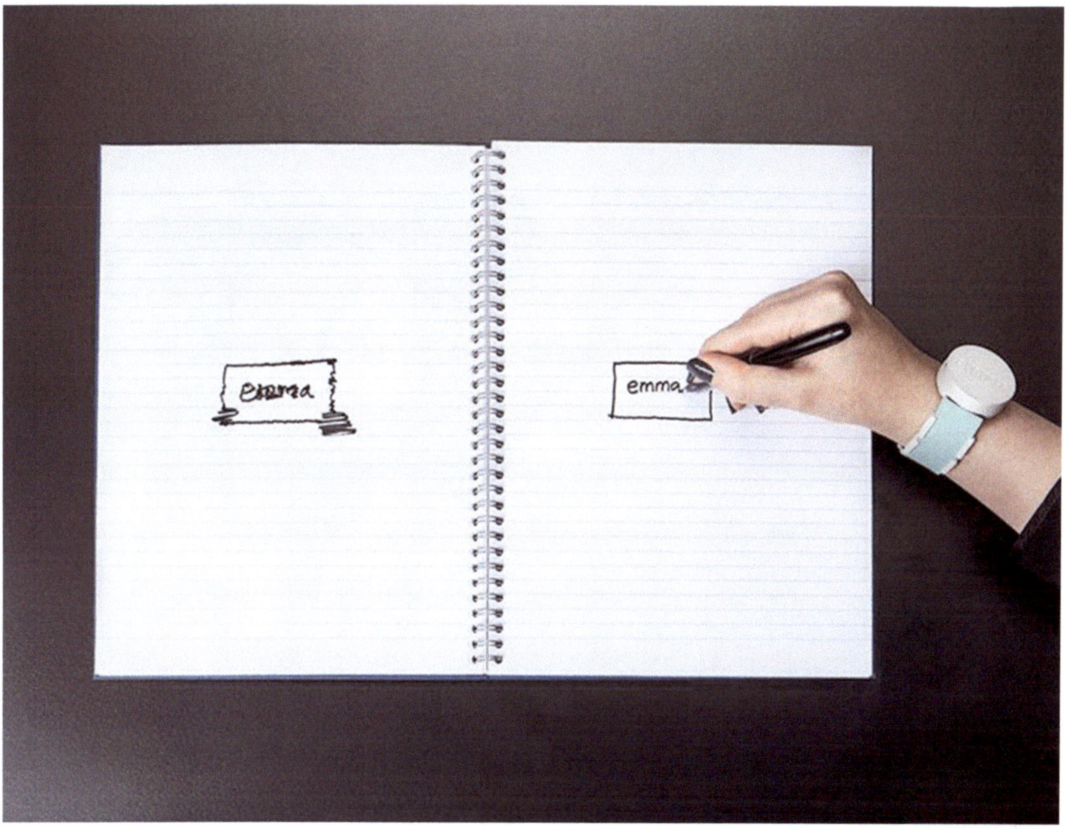

Fig. 3.3 Project Emma is designed by Emma Lawton and funded by Microsoft Research ("Project Emma" 2021)

Watch (EW) helps the person regain control of the hand in performing simple drawing and writing tasks: the device operates a rhythmic vibration effect using small motors around the wrist. A sensorimotor feedback loop regulates the ability to move, involving the perception of movement and body position.

The tremor could come due to an erroneous feedback loop, and then the brain overcompensates for an initial movement error, resulting in a continuous tremor. The submission of a vibrating signal by EW introduces to the user a white noise that can short-circuit the feedback loop, interrupting brains from sensing the initial error and continuing to try to overcome it.

The first concept of Emma Watch in 2017 was funded and developed by Microsoft Research Innovation in Cambridge, becoming Microsoft's Project Emma and entailing an increase in resources including the power of AI, the cloud, and machine learning to support a smart device that detects and counteracts the symptoms of PD ("Project Emma" 2021).

Gyroglove

Gyroglove is an assistive device for PD patients aiming to stabilize and improve the general hand movements of the person (Fig. 3.4). It is equipped with a miniature, dynamically adjustable gyroscope, positioned on the back of the hand within a case attached to the glove. When the device is switched on, the battery-powered gyroscope activates, and its orientation is adjusted by a precession hinge and turntable, both controlled by a small circuit board, then pushing back against the wearer's movements as the gyroscope tries to right itself ("GyroGloveTM|GyroGear". Accessed 2021).

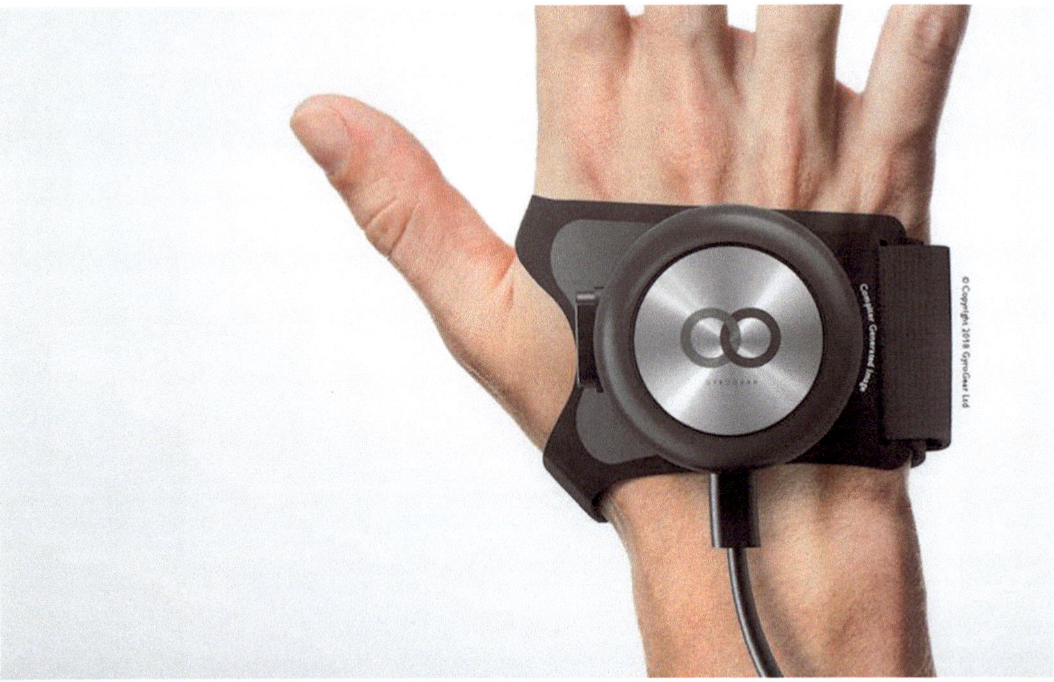

Fig. 3.4 GyroGlove was developed in 2014 by GyroGear and is based on a concept inspired by aerospace technology ("GyroGloveTM|GyroGear". Accessed 2021)

This device is based on a concept inspired by aerospace technology by the development team of engineers, designers, and medics of the GyroGear group, a medical device invention and development company based at Imperial College London. During its development the project won several prizes and awards thanks to its versatility: it is conceived to assist in activities like writing, eating, and everything that requires a specific hand ability. Gyroglove was developed in close contact with end users from the start, it was noticed that patients have difficulties optimally managing their medications, then during the experimentation the developers improved the tracking of tremors, detecting them each time the device is used, providing quantifiable data that will inform the users, their family but firstly their doctors, that can manage in a better way the prescription and dosage of medications thanks to a meticulous daily analysis of some aspects of the motor condition of the patient.

3.3 Conclusions

New technologies such as Artificial Intelligence, machine learning, Internet of Things, Big Data analysis, Virtual Reality, and others, are novel powerful tools for the design of products and services allowing the creation of devices and systems out of the traditional product categories typical of the healthcare field. Currently, technology can give new answers to people's needs, especially in prolonging the autonomous life of persons affected by degenerative impairments such as PD, providing them with a high quality of life.

The described devices are innovative significant samples of technology bringing new possibilities but requiring a deep study of systems' physical and cognitive ergonomics (Imbesi and Mincolelli 2020). The smart devices collected in this chapter were validated including the elderly with PD in the design processes, to observe their emotional attitude towards the devices' use, and to enhance their functional performances with selected technologies. The degree of usability of design projects addressed to older users should always consider their necessity to be as autonomous as possible in using proposed solutions, and not perceive them as medical devices for unhealthy diseased people.

Another aspect to focus on is that each product had an important impact on the silver market, we can hypothesize that one of the main reasons is the high degree of usability of the smart devices, all developed in contact with users from.

In the beginning; some of these design processes were defined by the relative companies as user-centered or human-centered but they all followed a very similar approach centered on the observation of the PD patient, firstly during his daily life to understand which are the needs whose satisfaction can really improve his quality of life, and then during the iterative process of the testing and improvement of the project.

References

T. Xu, J.B. Wendt, M. Potkonjak, Security of IoT systems: Design challenges and opportunities, in IEEE/ACM International Conference on Computer-Aided Design (ICCAD) **2014**, 417–423 (2014). https://doi.org/10.1109/ICCAD.2014.7001385

S. Borsci, S. Federici, Dall'interazione utente-tecnologia alla valutazione dell'usabilità: Una rassegna sullo stato dell'arte dei metodi e delle normative. G. Psicol. **2**, 233–253 (2008)

A. Rizzo, L'ergonomia Cognitiva, 1994, Accessed: Nov. 28, 2021. [Online]. Available: https://www.academia.edu/2678313/Lergonomia_Cognitiva

E. P. D. Association, The European Parkinson's Disease Standards of Care Consensus Statement. Accessed: Nov. 28, 2021. [Online]. Available: https://www.epda.eu.com/latest/resources/the-european-parkinsons-disease-standards-of-care-consensus-statement/

S. Imbesi and S. Scataglini, A User Centered Methodology for the Design of Smart Apparel for Older Users, *Sensors*, vol. 21, no. 8, Art. no. 8, 2021, https://doi.org/10.3390/s21082804.

T. L. Koreshoff, T. W. Leong, and T. Robertson, Approaching a human-centred internet of things, in *Proceedings of the 25th Australian Computer-Human Interaction Conference: Augmentation, Application, Innovation, Collaboration*, in OzCHI '13. New York, NY, USA: Association for Computing Machinery, 2013, pp. 363–366. https://doi.org/10.1145/2541016.2541093.

World Health Organization, *World report on ageing and health*. World Health Organization, 2015. Accessed: Nov. 27, 2021. [Online]. Available: https://apps.who.int/iris/handle/10665/186463

R. Thomson, J.L. Martin, S. Sharples, The psycho-social impact of home use medical devices on the lives of older people: a qualitative study. BMC Health Serv. Res. **13**(1), 467 (2013). https://doi.org/10.1186/1472-6963-13-467

D. Dorr et al., Informatics Systems to Promote Improved Care for Chronic Illness: A Literature Review. J. Am. Med. Inform. Assoc. JAMIA **14**(2), 156–163 (2007). https://doi.org/10.1197/jamia.M2255

N. Charness, G. Demiris, E. Krupinski, Designing Telehealth for an Aging Population: A Human Factors Perspective. Boca Raton: CRC Press (2011). https://doi.org/10.1201/b11229

R. Hurling et al., Using internet and mobile phone technology to deliver an automated physical activity program: randomized controlled trial. J. Med. Internet Res. **9**(2), e7 (2007). https://doi.org/10.2196/jmir.9.2.e7

S. Imbesi and G. Mincolelli, Monitoring Older People: An Overview of Devices Responding to Significant Needs of Elderly Affected by Parkinson's Disease, in *Advances in Additive Manufacturing, Modeling Systems and 3D Prototyping*, M. Di Nicolantonio, E. Rossi, and T. Alexander, Eds., in Advances in Intelligent Systems and Computing. Cham: Springer International Publishing, 2020, pp. 646–656. https://doi.org/10.1007/978-3-030-20216-3_60.

A. Pollini, G. A. Giacobone, and M. Zannoni, Aging and Interaction: Designing for Active Living Experiences, in *Internet of Things for Human-Centered Design: Application to Elderly Healthcare*, S. Scataglini, S. Imbesi, and G. Marques, Eds., in Studies in Computational Intelligence. , Singapore: Springer Nature, 2022, pp. 39–61. https://doi.org/10.1007/978-981-16-8488-3_3.

G. Mincolelli, M. Marchi, and S. Imbesi, Inclusive Design for Ageing People and the Internet of Things: Understanding Needs, in *Advances in Design for Inclusion*, G. Di Bucchianico and P. F. Kercher, Eds., in Advances in Intelligent Systems and Computing. Cham: Springer International Publishing, 2018, pp. 98–108. https://doi.org/10.1007/978-3-319-60597-5_9.

Emily, PKG (Personal Kinetigraph): Helping my Parkinson's Disease patients, Open Access Government. Accessed: Sep. 12, 2023. [Online]. Available: https://www.openaccessgovernment.org/pkg-personal-kinetigraph-helping-my-parkinsons-disease-patients/149244/

R. Pahwa, S.H. Isaacson, D. Torres-Russotto, F.B. Nahab, P.M. Lynch, K.E. Kotschet, Role of the Personal KinetiGraph in the routine clinical assessment of Parkinson's disease: recommendations from an expert panel. Expert Rev. Neurother. **18**(8), 669–680 (2018). https://doi.org/10.1080/14737175.2018.1503948

Path Finder|Innovative Walking Aid For Parkinson's Disease, Walk With Path. Accessed: Sep. 12, 2023. [Online]. Available: https://www.walkwithpath.com/pages/path-finder-for-professionals

H. Davis, Parkinson's disease: how a new device is helping patients to keep walking, *The Guardian*, 2018. Accessed: Nov. 28, 2021. [Online]. Available: https://www.theguardian.com/business-to-business/2018/oct/09/parkinsons-disease-how-device-helping-patients-to-keep-walking

Project Emma, Microsoft Research. Accessed: Nov. 28, 2021. [Online]. Available: https://www.microsoft.com/en-us/research/project/project-emma/

GyroGlove™|GyroGear. Accessed: Nov. 28, 2021. [Online]. Available: https://gyrogear.co/gyroglove

Design of a Smart mHealth System

4

Abstract

In this chapter, the author presents the process leading to the choice of the specific research field of the PASSO project. After explaining the general project requirements, the author considers the importance of the collection and classification of users' needs in this typology of design research. Moreover, it was defined the use case study of Gait Tutor as the starting point of this project: this reference can be implemented thanks to a different use of signals submitted to the users, specifically, it was considered to design novel sensory cues, requiring a low level of cognitive engagement, to influence the patient's gait and posture without making him feel overwhelmed. Finally, it was described the design process structure, composed of three cycles, each one divided in several design phases.

4.1 Research Project Definition

The starting point of the project was to address the elderly suffering from one of the different typologies of Dementia. To better identify the project context, several research questions were defined. The answers to these questions led to the definition of the main project requirements (Fig. 4.1).

(1) What is the typology of patients on whom Design Research could have the greatest impact?

Considering the most diffused typologies of Dementia, patients affected by PD are the ones with the highest number of symptoms related to movement but not necessarily connected to a cognitive decline. Those people could take great advantage in terms of autonomy and independence from a device that helps them in performing daily activities.

(2) Considering older PD patients, which are the daily activities most affected by the movement impairments related to the pathology?

There are a lot of daily actions that make the person feel autonomous and self-sufficient. PD at its first stages causes troubles in managing limb movements: that condition negatively affects the ability to perform daily easy tasks and makes the person feel frustrated and non-self-sufficient, causing important emotional repercussions. The most significant analyzed areas are the one of eating and the one of walking.

(3) Are there any products that already help older people affected by PD in eating and/or walking? Are those devices diffused? Do users appreciate those devices?

S. Imbesi, *Inclusive Design of a Smart Device for People with Parkinson's Disease*, Design For Inclusion 4, https://doi.org/10.1007/978-3-031-58249-3_4

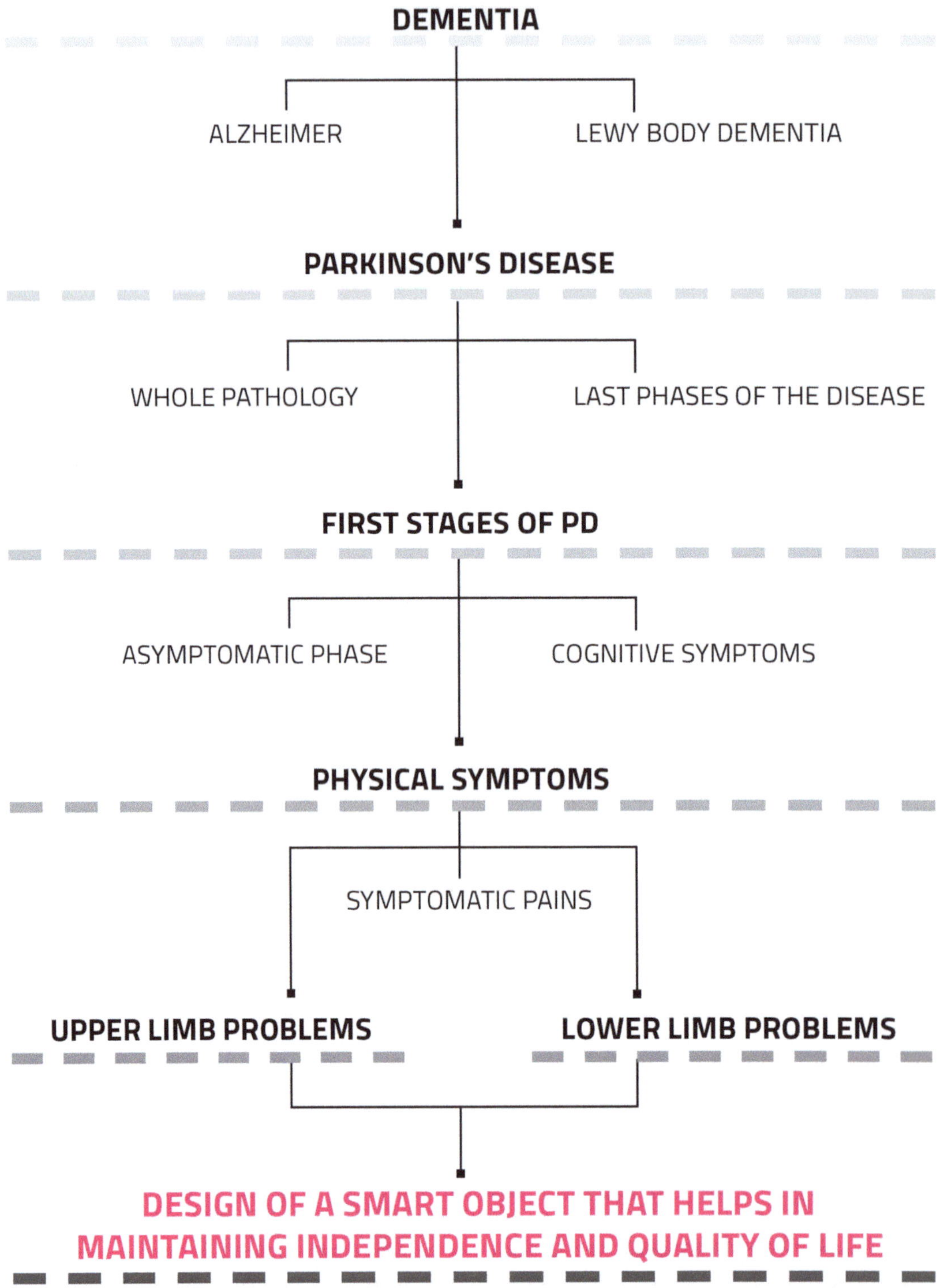

Fig. 4.1 Schematization of steps to the design project

There is a huge number of prototypes and smart products on the silver market, designed to help the elderly in performing daily activities like eating and walking.

The analysis took into consideration devices related to the Internet of Things with the primary function of monitoring the person in the short, medium, and long term for evaluations regarding the progression of the pathology. It was noticed that the most important problem in the diffusion of those products is the low level of usability and user-friendliness, which makes the user feel uncomfortable and ignore the advantages brought by the device.

(4) Which requirements should satisfy a smart device that helps older users in the walk monitoring the gait?

To design a device that can be effective in helping walking and monitoring the gait, it should:

- not a medical device but something different that doesn't remind users of the pathology they are affected by.
- provide data related to movements and postures, through the constant monitoring of the person.
- give immediate feedback to the user on its utility.
- be usable by the user on his own without the help of another person.
- not be abandoned after being used only a few times.

Project Requirements

Three aspects must necessarily be examined in an inclusive approach: the product itself and its technology, the people involved, and the environment in which it is to be used. Each of these three factors has a great complexity and heterogeneity within it (Tosi and Rinaldi 2015). The author decided to focus on a device that helps the older user making the person feel autonomous and not overwhelmed by impairments related to Parkinson's Disease.

The most important issues resulting from the previous analysis, to be developed in the research project were:

- The device/system doesn't provide medical evaluations and its functions are not related to the medical environment. It can be used even by the older person in his own house for short and long-term evaluations based on data detected by the smart device.
- The user needs to have immediate feedback on the device's utility, to use it frequently, and to optimize the detection of data related to his habits and performances.
- The device needs to be wearable or usable by the user himself without external help. It aims to give a sense of autonomy, so the device must be user-friendly, with a natural interface and intuitive controls, to avoid frustrations related to the low level of usability.

4.2 Research Project Technologies

Technologies currently available are making it possible to imagine better devices and environments for the assessment and monitoring of diseases like PD that involve the detection of the person's movement (Gibb and Lees 1988).

Patients affected by PD have specific needs, some of them are common to all aging people regardless of the pathologies they are affected by, and some others are distinctive of their disease. The products try to give solutions to some of those specific needs related to typical symptoms of Parkinson's disease.

The wearable devices that are currently designed for medical purposes, are tiny and comfortable, allowing patients to wear them with ease in their daily lives and making data collection especially convenient. The collection and use of data detected by inertial sensors and the emergence of Big Data have made possible the analysis and interpretation of enormous sets of data and information gathered by wearable devices. Compared to the large, complex machines previously used to collect information about movements associated with Parkinson's disease, today's wearable devices give a lot of advantages being less intrusive and without looking like medical devices, with the possibility to be purchased and used directly by the user without the intervention of medical personnel. Furthermore, the use of machine learning allows us to analyze the massive amounts of longitudinal data that can be gathered from wearable devices.

Smart Cues for PD

Smart systems using biofeedback seem to be a promising strategy for the mitigation of impairments brought by PD (Bega et al. 2014). Usually, these systems include smart wearables enabling sensory acquisition and triggering information thanks to cues (Sweeney et al. 2019). They work detecting gait-related parameters, such as a cadence modification or a change of oscillation, and, once detected several motor behaviors, can deliver proprioceptive cues (Martens et al. 2013). Smart systems using biofeedback allow the person with PD to improve freedom of movement and, consequently, autonomy and quality of life (Espay et al. 2016). Generally, stimuli used by cues are vibrotactile, visual, or auditory, providing the user with spatiotemporal information aiming to ease movements' initiation and continuation (Nieuwboer 2008).

At the moment, most of the existing scientific literature is about projects investigating the application of biofeedback to FOG, but it seems promising to analyze their impact on balance improvement and fall prevention (Cassimatis et al. 2016)–(Casamassima et al. 2014); these three are the main motor areas where sensory cues can be applied for the improvement of PD users' motor abilities.

Biofeedback systems are generally composed of an actuation system providing cueing, a sensory system acquiring physiological and physical measurements, and a processing unit collecting, processing, and controlling data related to the actuation system when necessary (Gonçalves et al. 2021). The sensory system integrates Inertial Measurement Units (IMU) into the smart device.

Biofeedback systems have two main objectives: preserving the patient's optimal gait and posture, preventing postural imbalances, falls, and FOG, and improving rescue strategies when gait worsening has occurred (Rossi-Izquierdo et al. 2013). From the preserving perspective, smart cues have the role of stabilizing balance, thanks to the submission of biofeedback aimed to improve gait and posture parameters related to balance (Nanhoe-Mahabier et al. 2012). Otherwise, in the perspective of improvement of rescue strategies for onset impairments, these smart systems have the replacement role of providing sensory cues, in substitution of the person's sensory abilities, to facilitate motor response generation (Punin et al. 2017).

Currently, no systems are integrating all components in a single smart device to improve its usability, this kind of design would put in the same location sensors and actuators avoiding intrusiveness and heaviness. More studies are still requested to understand precisely how every sensory cue should be submitted and to which motor condition cues should be applied (Sweeney et al. 2019).

Considering that, as said before, the cues submission can be used to manage FOG or balance control and risk of fall, it was decided to work on balance control where considered variables are body sway metrics, as the limit of stability (LOS), position error (PE), center of position (CoP) path length, CoP velocity and roll/ pitch sway angle (High et al. 2018).

Users' Needs About Technology

The needs analysis was carried out in different steps at the beginning where many contributors used surveys, direct interviews, focus groups, and others. Then, information was elaborated to obtain brief statements that could express the requirements deduced by the different categories of users involved in the project. These statements were classified depending on the user that expressed them, on the field they were related to, and on the relevance they had for the design of smart devices (Mincolelli et al. 2018).

In the first part of the research, thanks to scientific literature, direct observation, and some talk with users and medical staff members, it has been analyzed the context and the general requirements of the chosen user figures. The objective of this phase was to discover important needs to identify a product typology that could be useful to solve specific problems or to find a daily problematic situation that could be solved with an innovative device not belonging to the existing types.

The major problems encountered concerned activities related to the motor sector, specifically the sphere of ambulation, and physical activities involving handwork, like autonomous food consumption. It was chosen to focus on the design of solutions for the improvement of safe autonomous walking, to make the older person more confident and independent, delaying the user's necessity for walking aids.

The objective of the survey was to focus on the reasons for the satisfaction and/or frustration of the respondents about certain actions in daily life. The collected information has been translated into users' needs, expressed with the peculiar language of the people they belong to. An alphanumeric code has been assigned to each need, to classify it according to the source and to the person it concerns (Imbesi et al. 2021).

4.3 Case Study: Gait Tutor

The project starts as an implementation of the Gait Tutor (GT) project ("Rehabilitation - Gait Tutor", mHealth Technologies. 2021), a gait monitoring system born from a collaboration between the Engineering Department of the University of Bologna, the Istituto delle Scienze Neurologiche di Bologna and the company mHealth Technologies. It was developed to provide gait training to people with PD outside specialized centers through a virtual assistant (via real-time vocal feedback on gait performance).

The system consists of inertial measurement units (IMUs), a Smartphone, and a dedicated app that can process the IMU data in real time (Ferrari et al. 2016) (Fig. 4.2). It can provide feedback to the user to help him improve their walking as if a therapist were walking next to the patient (e.g. when indicated, the app says: "Take the longest stride"). GT is a certified medical device that is now commercialized by mHealth Technologies, a startup that was created as a spinoff of the University of Bologna ("Rehabilitation—Gait Tutor", mHealth Technologies. 2021). GT has an interface on the smartphone and can connect automatically to two wearable sensors on the shoes and one in the chest.

By analyzing in real-time the walking pattern of the patient, it can provide vocal feedback to improve walking (Casamassima et al. 2014). Different characteristics of walking can be trained (e.g. stride length, gait speed, posture during walking, and so on). So, gait training can be performed anytime, anywhere. The training set-up can be modified remotely by clinicians and be used as a form of telerehabilitation. The results of the walking training (e.g. number of sessions, distance walked, average gait speed) can also be accessed remotely by clinicians. GT is therefore ready to be used in a tele-rehabilitation setting.

Possibilities of Implementation with Design

The current version of the GT system uses vocal instructions to encourage the user to modify several aspects of the gait. It was possible to observe that this kind of communication involves significantly the persons' cognitive abilities asking for a high degree of concentration, taking the risk of making the user feel overwhelmed by the multitasking activity. From this consideration, it was evaluated to start the design process using UCD methodologies to design and test sensory cues, involving different sensory channels (one or more at a time), to observe and evaluate how different typologies of cues impact the person's gait. The involved senses were hearing, sight, and touch. Auditory

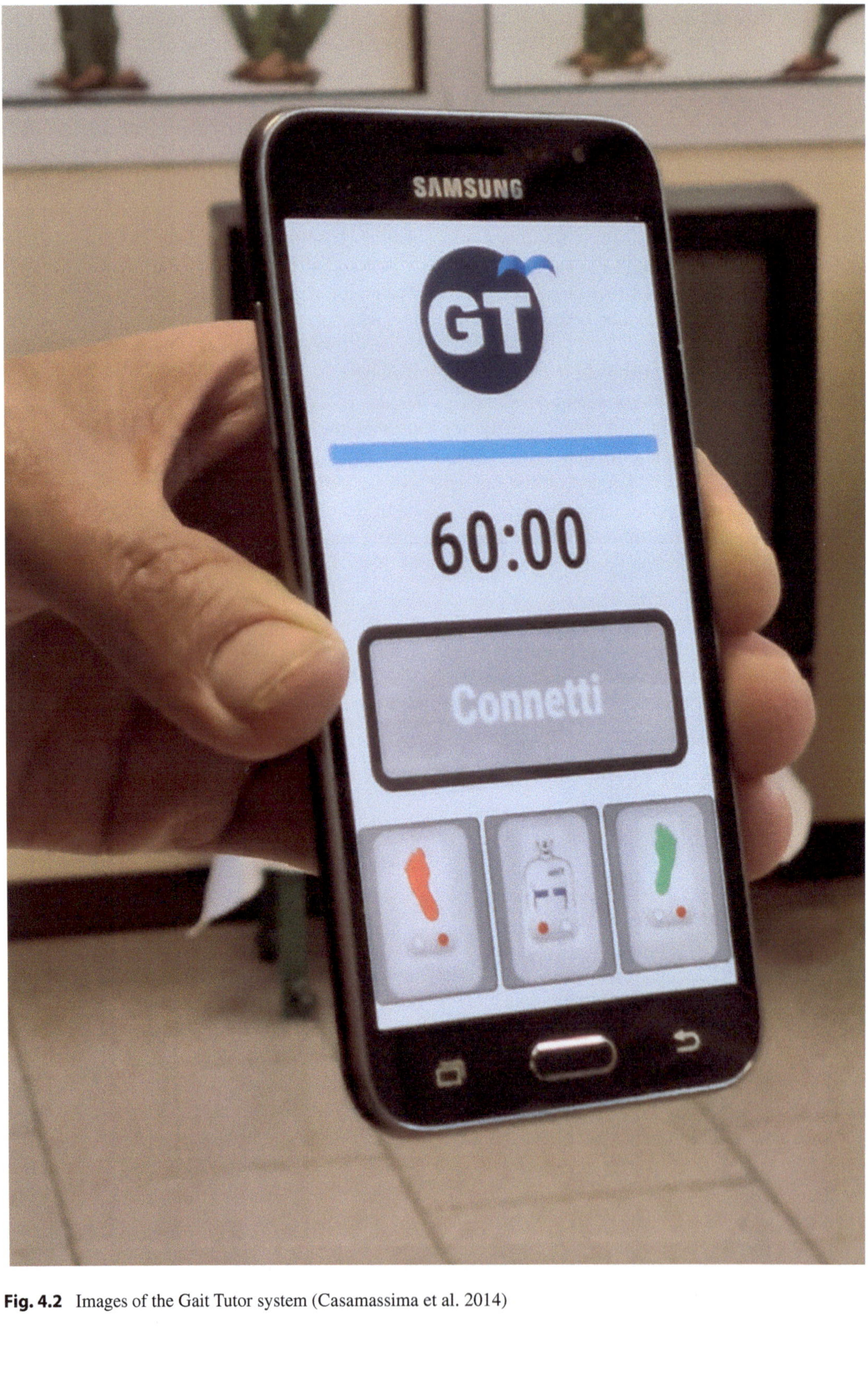

Fig. 4.2 Images of the Gait Tutor system (Casamassima et al. 2014)

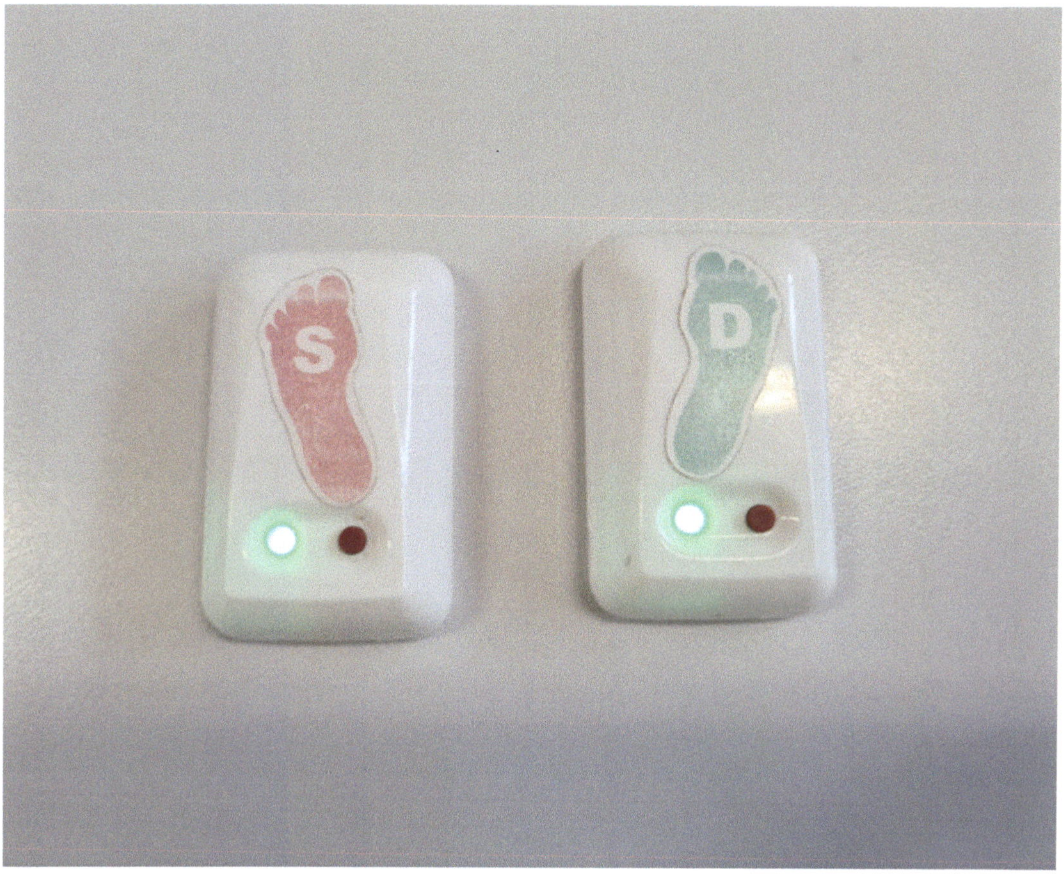

Fig. 4.2 (continued)

cues were submitted by earphones (as in GT), while visual and vibratory by Smart Glasses.

This first stage of the project aimed to acquire knowledge about cues for the realization of a smart wearable device, able to provide the person with PD with a training and tele rehabilitation system, specifically designed to answer the user's needs (Imbesi 2022). The current GT system uses sensor devices on the user's shoes to monitor the gait, a belt on the chest to monitor the posture and a Smartphone with earphones as actuators (Fig. 4.3). The following stage of the project was the development of a wearable device integrated with the GT system, merging sensors and actuators to gain a higher degree of usability and wearability to improve the person's training experience (Figs. 4.4and 4.5).

The last part of the project was the development of the graphical interface of the web application managing the system. This part of the project output was expected to significantly influence the user in the perception of the whole project.

4.4 Research Project Structure

In light of the previously analyzed UC methodologies, considering the complexity and multidisciplinarity of the project, it was decided to follow the UCD design process composed of the phases of planning (P1), analyzing (P2), creating (P3), and verifying (P4) (User-Centered Design Process Map. 2023). This approach is supposed to help in managing and simplifying the design process.

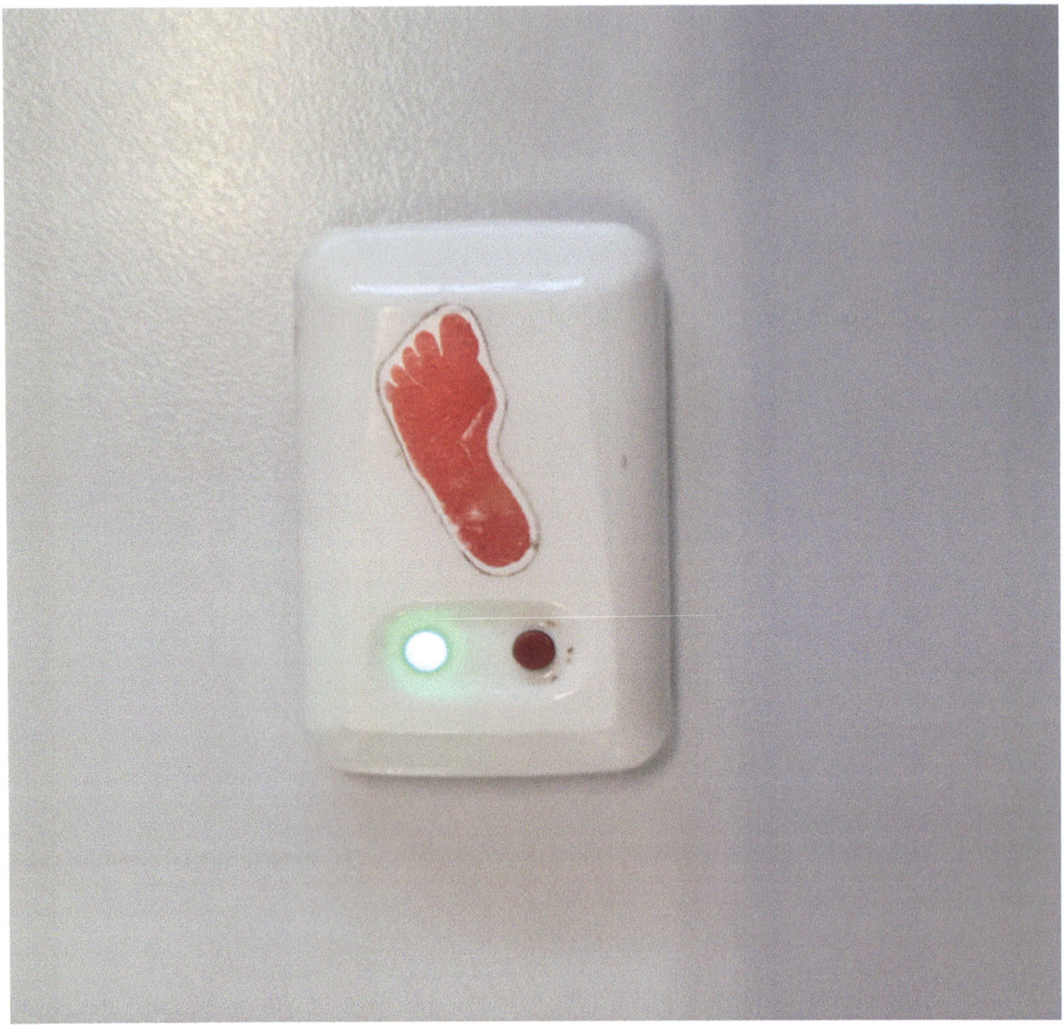

Fig. 4.2 (continued)

Considering the design of a mHealth system using sensory cues as the aim of the PASSO project, it was decided to define which were the main components that were going to be designed and developed (Imbesi 2022). Three main elements were identified: the sensory cues submitted by the system, the wearable device submitting the designed cues, and, finally, the digital interface allowing users to manage the system. Moreover, it was considered to structure the project considering each element of the system to be designed as an autonomous design cycle, composed of the previously mentioned four phases.

This structure is supposed to improve the project results as it will allow the application of the steps uc to the design of each element, refining the objectives and adapting the methodology to them. Moreover, the results of each cycle will serve as input to the next cycle but will also be considered autonomously. Each cycle can be deepened through its iteration until satisfactory results are obtained (Fig. 4.5).

The three cycles panned are:

Cycle 1 (C1): Sensory cues and system.

Cycle 2 (C2): Devices submitting sensory cues.

Cycle 3 (C3): Interfaces for PD users.

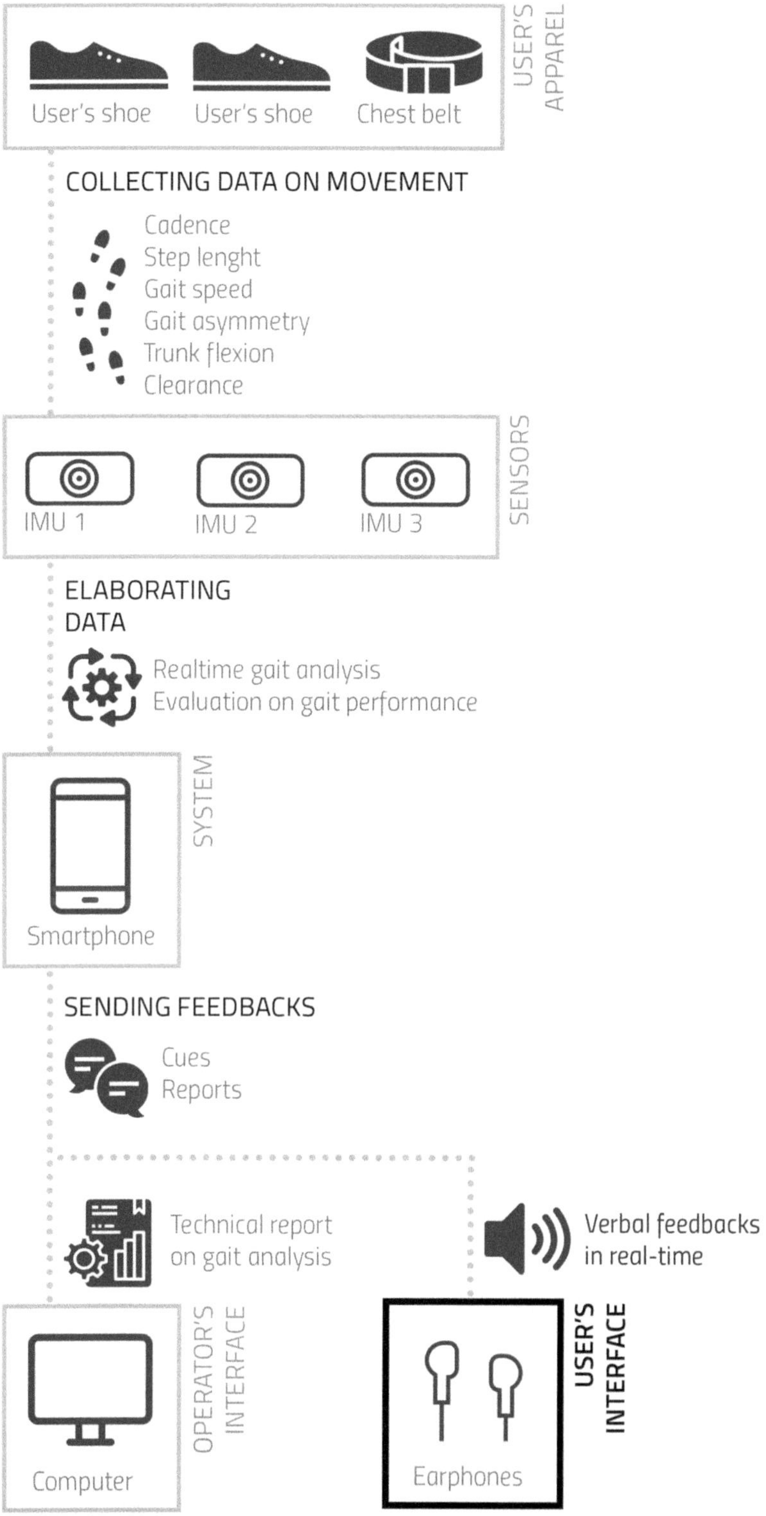

Fig. 4.3 Scheme representing the system of Gait Tutor. The system collects data on movement, elaborates data, and then sends feedback to the user thanks to earphones

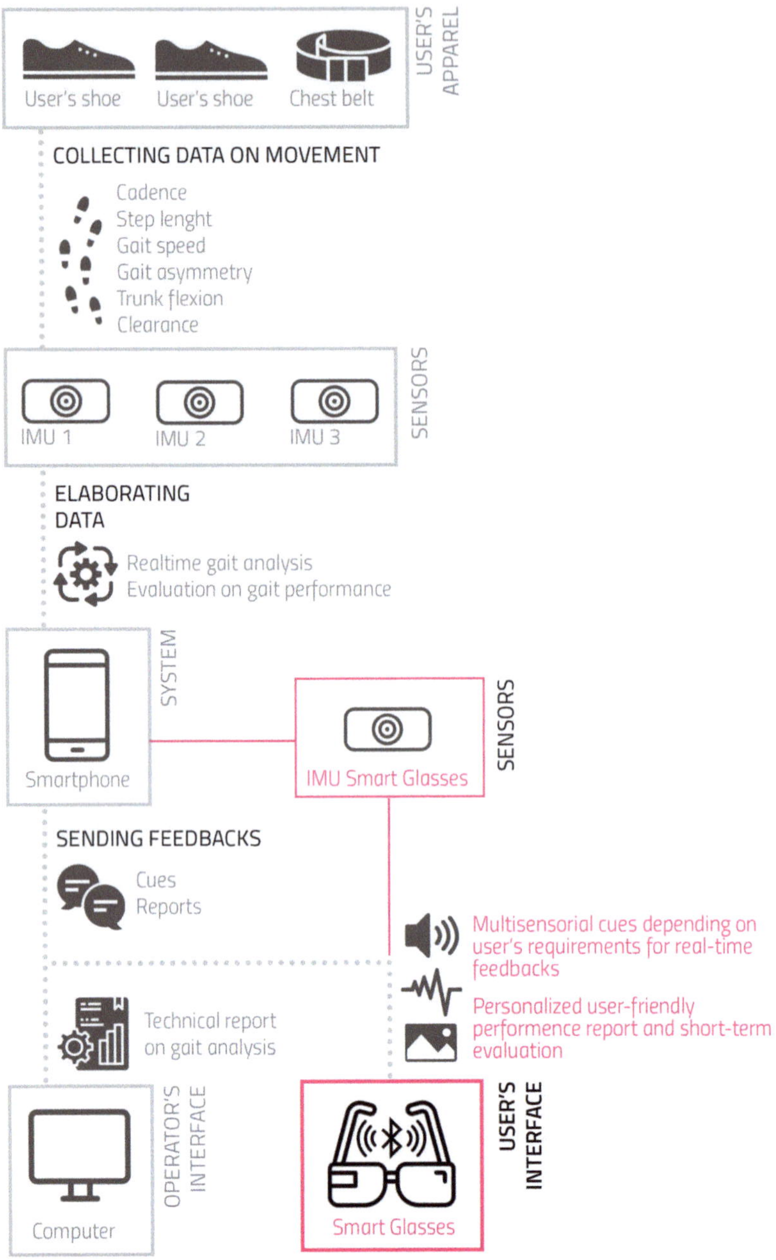

Fig. 4.4 Scheme representing the short-term hypothesis of improvement of Gait Tutor. The Smart Glasses are integrated into the system, their IMUs provide the system with additional information and the lenses offer images giving new feedback to the user

Project Image

The chosen name for the research project was PASSO (PA rkinson's Smart Sensory-cues for Olders). The project logotype was inspired by sensory channels involved in the design project.

The chosen typeface was simple and easily interpretable.

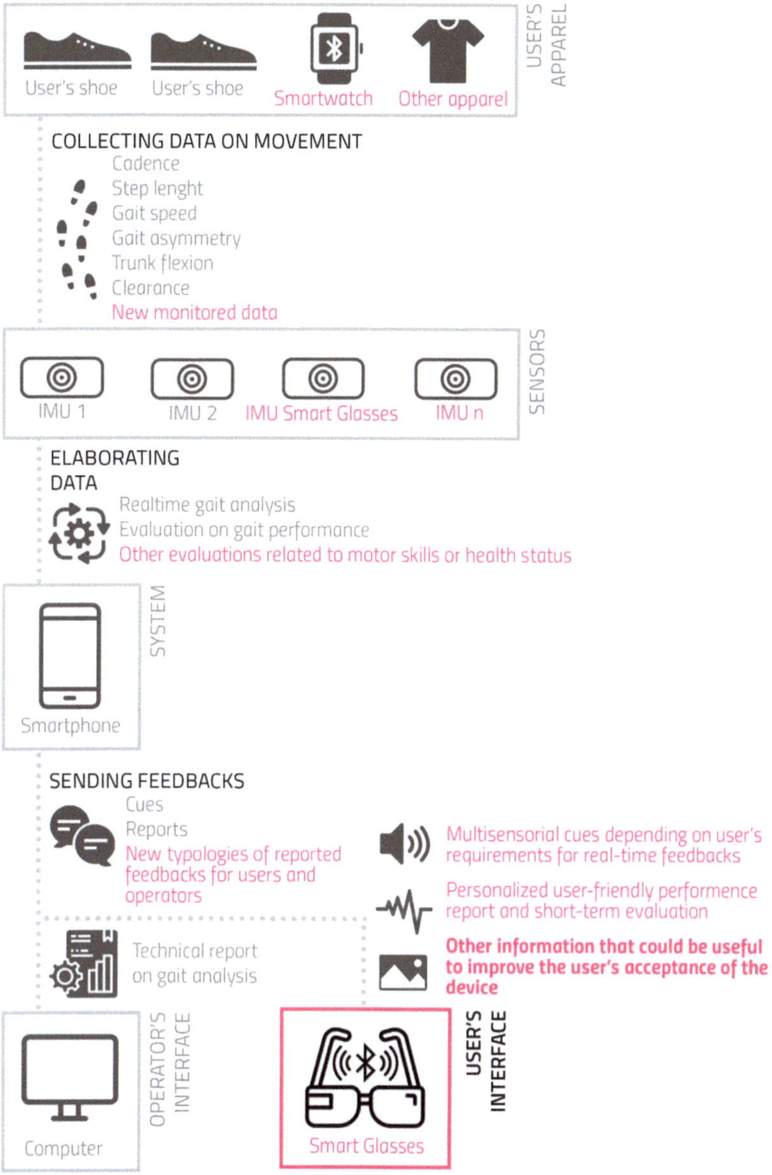

Fig. 4.5 Scheme representing the long-term hypothesis of improvement of Gait Tutor. The system is scalable and several smart devices are integrated into the system, their IMUs provide the system information about different parameters of the person. Feedback to the user is submitted by Smart Glasses or other kinds of devices, preferably merging sensors and actuators

Chosen colors are black, white, grey, and magenta, to have a high degree of color contrast and be able to distinguish the different components (Figs. 4.6 and 4.7).

4.5 Conclusions

The design research project's adjective was defined through some research questions identifying the context of healthcare smart devices for

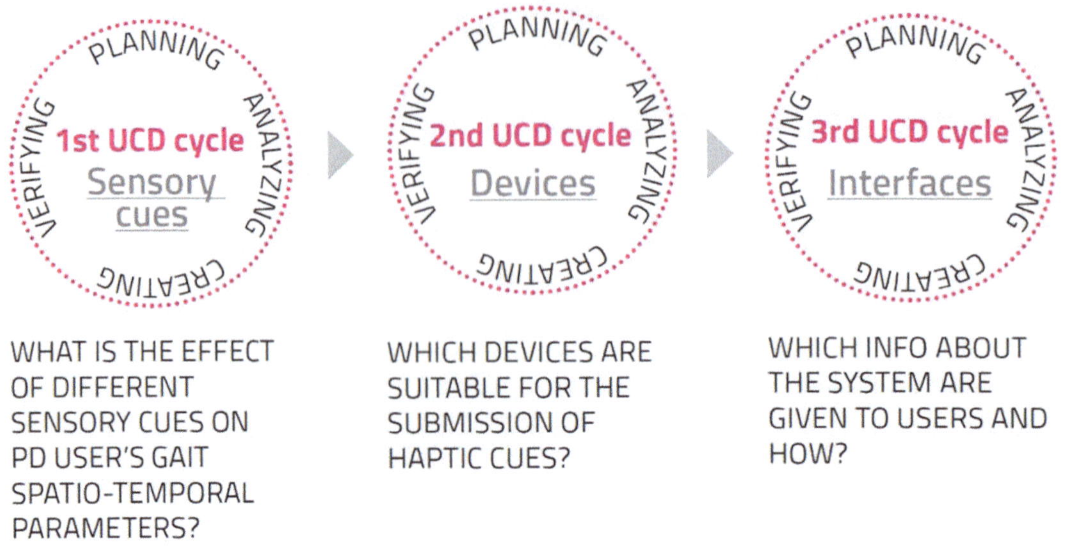

Fig. 4.6 Schematization of the three cycles of the project, each one composed of four phases: Planning, Analyzing, Creating, and Verifying

Fig. 4.7 Logotype versions

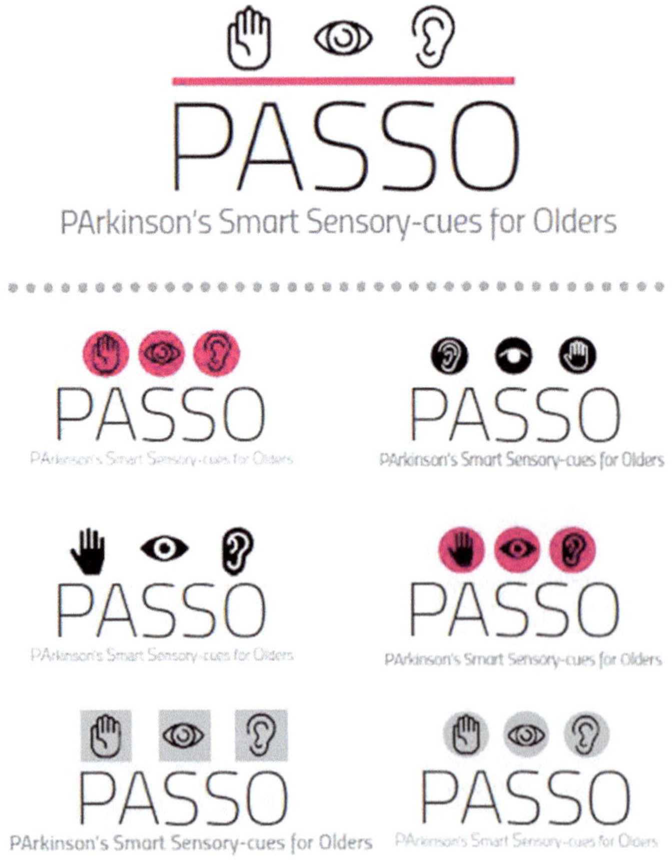

the rehabilitation of motor capabilities of people with PD. The rehabilitation system is supposed to provide sensory feedback to patients needing to correct their gait and postural behavior.

Users facing the degeneration brought by PD have peculiar requirements that should be deeply analyzed to be satisfied, the project plans to apply methodological strategies to improve the outputs' usability and accessibility.

The PASSO research project starts as the implementation of the commercial Gait Tutor system, conceived to provide users with instructions about walking performance thanks to vocal advices.

References

F. Tosi, A. Rinaldi, *Il design per l'Home Care. L'approccio Human-Centred Design nel progetto dei dispositivi medici*. Firenze: Dip. di Architettura (2015)

W.R. Gibb, A.J. Lees, The relevance of the Lewy body to the pathogenesis of idiopathic Parkinson's disease. J. Neurol. Neurosurg. Psychiatry **51**(6), 745–752 (1988). https://doi.org/10.1136/jnnp.51.6.745

D. Bega, P. Gonzalez-Latapi, C. Zadikoff, T. Simuni, A review of the clinical evidence for complementary and alternative therapies in Parkinson's disease. Curr. Treat. Options. Neurol. **16**(10), 314 (2014). https://doi.org/10.1007/s11940-014-0314-5

D. Sweeney, L. R. Quinlan, P. Browne, M. Richardson, P. Meskell, G. ÓLaighin, A technological review of wearable cueing devices addressing freezing of gait in Parkinson's disease, *Sensors*, 19(6), 6 (2019). https://doi.org/10.3390/s19061277

K.A.E. Martens, F. Pieruccini-Faria, Q.J. Almeida, Could sensory mechanisms be a core factor that underlies freezing of gait in Parkinson's disease? PLoS ONE **8**(5), e62602 (2013). https://doi.org/10.1371/journal.pone.0062602

A.J. Espay et al., Technology in Parkinson's disease: Challenges and opportunities. Mov. Disord. off. J. Mov. Disord. Soc. **31**(9), 1272–1282 (2016). https://doi.org/10.1002/mds.26642

A. Nieuwboer, Cueing for freezing of gait in patients with Parkinson's disease: a rehabilitation perspective. Mov. Disord. off. J. Mov. Disord. Soc. **23**(2), S475-481 (2008). https://doi.org/10.1002/mds.21978

C. Cassimatis, K.P.Y. Liu, P. Fahey, M. Bissett, The effectiveness of external sensory cues in improving functional performance in individuals with Parkinson's disease: a systematic review with meta-analysis. Int. J. Rehabil. Res. **39**(3), 211–218 (2016). https://doi.org/10.1097/MRR.0000000000000171

H.R. Gonçalves, A.M. Rodrigues, C.P. Santos, Vibrotactile biofeedback devices in Parkinson's disease: a narrative review. Med. Biol. Eng. Comput. **59**(6), 1185–1199 (2021). https://doi.org/10.1007/s11517-021-02365-3

F. Casamassima, A. Ferrari, B. Milosevic, P. Ginis, E. Farella, L. Rocchi, A wearable system for gait training in subjects with Parkinson's disease, *Sensors*, 14(4), 4 (2014). https://doi.org/10.3390/s140406229

M. Rossi-Izquierdo et al., Vibrotactile neurofeedback balance training in patients with Parkinson's disease: Reducing the number of falls. Gait Posture **37**(2), 195–200 (2013). https://doi.org/10.1016/j.gaitpost.2012.07.002

W. Nanhoe-Mahabier, J.H. Allum, E.P. Pasman, S. Overeem, B.R. Bloem, The effects of vibrotactile biofeedback training on trunk sway in Parkinson's disease patients. Parkinsonism Relat. Disord. **18**(9), 1017–1021 (2012). https://doi.org/10.1016/j.parkreldis.2012.05.018

C. Punin, B. Barzallo, M. Huerta, A. Bermeo, M. Bravo, L. Carlos, *Wireless devices to restart walking during an episode of FOG on patients with Parkinson's disease* (2017), p. 6. https://doi.org/10.1109/ETCM.2017.8247520

C.M. High, H.F. McHugh, S.C. Mills, S. Amano, J.E. Freund, S. Vallabhajosula, Vibrotactile feedback alters dynamics of static postural control In persons with Parkinson's disease but not older adults at high fall risk. Gait Posture **63**, 202–207 (2018). https://doi.org/10.1016/j.gaitpost.2018.05.010

G. Mincolelli, M. Marchi, and S. Imbesi, Inclusive design for ageing people and the internet of things: Understanding needs, in *Advances in Design for Inclusion*, G. Di Bucchianico and P. F. Kercher, Eds., in Advances in Intelligent Systems and Computing (Cham: Springer International Publishing, 2018), pp. 98–108. https://doi.org/10.1007/978-3-319-60597-5_9

S. Imbesi, G. Mincolelli, F. Petrocchi, How to enhance aging people's wellness by means of human centered and co-design methodology, in *Advances in Simulation and Digital Human Modeling*, D. N. Cassenti, S. Scataglini, S. L. Rajulu, and J. L. Wright, Eds., in Advances in Intelligent Systems and Computing (Cham: Springer International Publishing, 2021), pp. 216–225. https://doi.org/10.1007/978-3-030-51064-0_28

Rehabilitation—Gait Tutor, mHealth Technologies. Accessed: Nov. 28, 2021. [Online]. Available: https://mhealthtechnologies.it/products-wearable-sensors-smartphone-apps/rehabilitation-gait-tutor/

A. Ferrari, P. Ginis, A. Nieuwboer, R. Greenlaw, A. Muddiman, L. Chiari, Handling Gait Impairments of Persons with Parkinson's Disease by Means of Real-Time Biofeedback in a Daily Life Environment, in *Inclusive Smart Cities and Digital Health*, C. K. Chang, L. Chiari, Y. Cao, H. Jin, M. Mokhtari, and H. Aloulou, Eds., in Lecture Notes in Computer Science (Cham: Springer International Publishing, 2016), pp. 250–261. https://doi.org/10.1007/978-3-319-39601-9_22

S. Imbesi, Human-centered design for older users: A design methodology for the development of smart devices and systems related to health care, in *Internet of Things for Human-Centered Design: Application to Elderly Healthcare*, S. Scataglini, S. Imbesi, and G. Marques, Eds., in Studies in Computational Intelligence (Singapore: Springer Nature, 2022), pp. 25–37. https://doi.org/10.1007/978-981-16-8488-3_2

User-Centered Design Process Map. Accessed: Sep. 19, 2023. [Online]. Available: https://www.usability.gov/how-to-and-tools/resources/ucd-map.html

5 Cycle 1: Smart Sensory Cues

Abstract

The first design cycle of the PASSO project aims to design and test sensory cues using the visual, auditory, and tactile channels to suggest to the user how to positively modify the gait and posture. This chapter describes the four phases of planning, analyzing, creating, and verifying. The planning phase defines users and context; the analyzing one studies users' requirements given by people about their perception of sensory cues, and technical constraints from available technologies influencing choices about smart devices; the creating phase regards the design and development of visual, auditive, and vibratory cues' prototypes; and, finally, the verifying phase is about the validation of the designed solutions thanks to a testing protocol with the involvement of several users.

5.1 Structure of Cycle 1

As described in the previous chapter, the PASSO project followed an iterative design process composed of cycles consisting of several phases, following a User-Centered (UCD) methodology to set the design process (User-Centered Design Process Map 2023).

The research project identified four design phases described as:

- planning phase (P1): describing context, objectives, and resources;
- analyzing phase (P2): studying users and technologies related to the project;
- creating phase (P3): defining the design and the prototypes to be tested;
- verifying phase (P4): testing the developed solutions involving users.

Moreover, three cycles and related aims were planned each one developing a specific part of the overall research project:

- Cycle 1 (C1): Sensory cues and the system managing them;
- Cycle 2 (C2): Devices submitting sensory cues;
- Cycle 3 (C3): System interfaces for users.

This chapter describes the development of the first design cycle from the Design Research perspective, focusing on the defined design methodologies and the followed design process. Specifically, the first design cycle aimed at the design of sensory cues and the mHealth system used to validate the adopted technology within the laboratory context in the presence of healthcare professionals and technicians. The multidisciplinary team tested a panel of different auditory, visual, and haptic cues, analyzing which sensory channels were most sensitive to which type of stimulation and which gait parameters were greatly influenced by this kind

S. Imbesi, *Inclusive Design of a Smart Device for People with Parkinson's Disease*, Design For Inclusion 4, https://doi.org/10.1007/978-3-031-58249-3_5

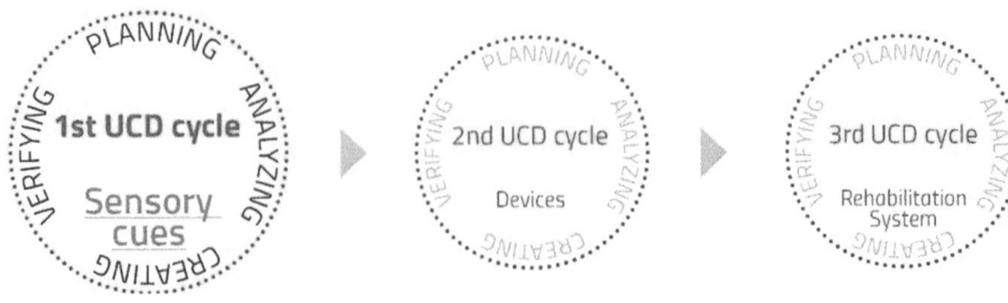

Fig. 5.1 Schematization of the UCD methodology, applied through iterative design cycles

of stimuli, implying a low cognitive involvement and better physical performance (Fig. 5.1) (Imbesi and Corzani 2023).

The project started as the Gait Tutor system implementation, which currently works with only the auditory channel by earphones. It would be desirable to innovate the system with more typologies of cues involving even other senses. The Gait Tutor system was considered a project invariant and was associated with devices able to submit different typologies of sensory cues.

5.2 Planning Phase (C1P1)

General project objectives and strategies guiding the overall design process were defined during the planning phase.

This first design cycle aimed to analyze how visual, auditory, and sensory cues submitted to the system's users, using the Gait Tutor system implemented with Smart Glasses (SG) and earphones, can influence people's gait.

A fundamental topic addressed in this cycle was the definition of which abilities were to be included in the team to gain project success. The multidisciplinary mix of skills and competencies identified as suitable to set objectives and process development comprised three leading professional figures (during the project development, depending on current necessities, the multidisciplinary team was enriched with professionals with specific competencies strictly related to the design phase):

- Designers (user research, usability, UCD methodology, interaction design, product design, visual design, etc.) to identify design strategies for the project development, engaging users in the design process;
- Technical operators (biomedical engineering, computer science and technology, informatics, etc.) to create the digital infrastructure for the system realization;
- Medical operators (neurology, physiatry, physiotherapy, geriatrics, etc.) participate in the definition of users' requirements and guide the experimentation with people.

Together with the cited professionals, even users were engaged to participate in the project's requirements definition and validate created solutions.

Once analyzed possibilities and limitations in the research project, the multidisciplinary team defined the design cycle's main research questions:

- Which images, sounds, and vibrations mostly influence gait speed, stride length, and cadence?
- Which are the ones stressing the user the least?
- Which ones induce the most immediate reaction?

Starting from the need to answer these questions, different sensory cues were specifically conceived and designed.

The results of this design phase, obtained by designing and selecting several signals for submission to users with or without Parkinson's disease (PD), were supposed to be the starting point for the following cycle.

Understanding the Context

As previously specified, the research project developed the design process of a system providing multimodal sensory cues for gait rehabilitation to people affected by Parkinson's Disease (PD).

The PASSO project was designed to be used on people with PD in ambulatory contexts and outside specialized centers to rehabilitate postural and transient gait disturbances and provide gait training at home, respectively.

Physical exercise and physiotherapy help overcome PD motor impairments by decelerating and postponing the unavoidable motor decline (Goodwin et al. 2008; Tomlinson et al. 2012). Moreover, scientific literature suggests that in the PD context, the effects of exercise can be enhanced by increasing subjects' cognitive engagement with practice, thanks to the submission of cueing or feedback (Petzinger et al. 2013). Cueing is a temporal or spatial sensory stimulus able to ease and facilitate repetitive movements by providing an explicit motor target.

Several scientific reviews indicate that various cueing modalities effectively influence the gait and health-related quality of life (Lim et al. 2005; Nieuwboer et al. 2007; Rochester et al. 2010; Rubinstein et al. 2002). Interestingly, recent advances in mobile technology have shown that augmented unisensory cues can even be applied to improve gait using wearable systems. Besides, less is noted about the possible benefits and usability of multisensory feedback (Rocha et al. 2014; Sánchez-Ferro and Maetzler 2016; Ayena et al. Oct. 2017).

For the definition of the operating context of the system, the author decided to consider the primary environment as the ambulatory, in the presence of a medical operator, and as a secondary environment, it was considered outdoor paths selected by the user.

5.3 Analyzing Phase (C1P2)

The analyzing phase considered human requirements and technical constraints and consisted of reviewing specific scientific literature, analyzing the systems operating with similar technologies and for analogous users state-of-the-art, and submitting interviews to representants of the categories of users involved in the project.

Users for Human Requirements

The developed system was conceived for PD subjects who are facing the initial or intermediate stages of the disease (Hoehn and Yahr scale: I-II), dealing with several issues but most of all with a physical decline affecting walking and motor skills in general, impacting functional independence, and well-being.

PD is defined as a neurologic disorder, the progressive degeneration of some typologies of cells leads the affected individual to the four cardinal symptoms of PD: tremors, rigidity, postural instability, and bradykinesia (Davie 2008). Cited symptoms characterize a large and various amount of physical impairments, some with a highly destructive effect specifically on physical abilities related to the gait (Nieuwboer et al. 2001). These gait impairments commonly lead to consider disabled people with PD (Capecci et al. 2014). This disease can cause gait instability and patterning difficulty with increased cadence, reduced stride length, freezing of gait, and reduced velocity. Although pharmacological therapies, gait impairments are persistent and are related to the significant reduction of the person's independence and personal safety, confirming the importance of developing alternative and innovative approaches and strategies to manage gait problems (Spaulding et al. 2013).

The analysis of users produced considerations on motor and cognitive performance related to the submission of sensory and multisensory cues for the empowerment and monitoring of gait performance. Considering motor dysfunctions correlated with PD, it is evident that personalized gait rehabilitation could facilitate patients' motor performance. In particular, improving gait slowness, variability, asymmetry, and even postural control (Peterson and Horak 2016).

Scientific literature assesses that the use of external sensory cues (e.g., auditory, visual, and haptic) to reinforce attention toward a specific task, is an effective gait-rehabilitation solution for persons with PD (Gonçalves et al. 2021; Tsai et al. 2020): the cues stimulate the voluntary executive component of the action thanks to the activation of attentional-executive motor control system and bypassing the dysfunctional, habitual, sensorimotor basal ganglia network (Ayena et al. Oct. 2017; Ferrazzoli et al. 2018; Wegen et al. 2014).

In the past, auditory cueing during gait has typically been provided continuously in an open loop (regardless of gait performance) (Rocha et al. 2014). In the therapeutic context, people were invited to match the foot movement's initiation or continuation (Lim et al. 2005). Recent innovations in wearables and mobile technology provide promising new ways to offer closed-loop feedback to people with PD during gait (Sánchez-Ferro and Maetzler 2016), which can overcome traditional open-loop cues, providing customized cueing: stimuli are triggered in real-time when gait deviates from normal, thus providing patients instant feedback on their performance.

In the sensory feedback field, proprioceptive cues (such as haptic stimuli) require little or no cognitive processing or attention (Peterson and Smulders 2015). Besides, a multi-sensory approach enhances perceptual processing, known to be reduced in PD subjects (Davidsdottir et al. 2005; Shams and Seitz 2008). Therefore, using a different combination of sensory inputs might significantly change the motor response's effectiveness and efficiency to the feedback. Thanks to advances in technology, visual feedback is feasible through Smart Glasses (SG) (Wiederhold 2013). SG seems to be a promising modality to give tailored signals and personal assistance to people with PD in their daily life.

Indeed, McNaney et al. found that participants with PD were generally positive about SG as an everyday assistive device; however, usability issues and social stigma still hinder its general acceptance.

Besides, considering the cognitive point of view, it was determined from the analysis that simulations should occur through cues that do not represent or pronounce the action to be performed, but rather try to induce it through intuitive and straightforward communication, not requiring cognitive or interpretative processing by the user (Peterson and Smulders 2015).

Technologies for Technical Constraints

To face typical gait problems generated by PD, recent advances in mobile technology have shown that augmented sensory feedback can help to improve walking (Rocha et al. 2014; Sánchez-Ferro and Maetzler 2016). An existing system for gait rehabilitation (Gait Tutor system) makes persons with PD better aware of their gait performance through augmented verbal feedback (Vuzix Blade® Upgraded Version, 2021).

Considering that the project started as an implementation of the Gait Tutor system, working using only the auditory channel thanks to earphones, it would be interesting to innovate the system with other typologies of cues involving more sense channels. The Gait Tutor system was assumed to project invariant, associating it with smart glasses (SG), able to submit other kinds of sensory cues.

Thanks to SG, real-time visual and haptic signals are also possible: the PASSO research project investigated strategies to design an innovative mHealth system obtained by integrating the smartphone-based Gait Tutor system with Android commercial smart glasses (Casamassima et al. 2014).

The Gait Tutor system was composed of a smartphone app that processes data streamed from the IMUs positioned on the user's shoes and elaborates gait parameters to trigger real-time verbal feedback impacting the gait. Innovatively, the smartphone app related to the Gait Tutor system was modified to allow information exchange via Bluetooth with SG. These

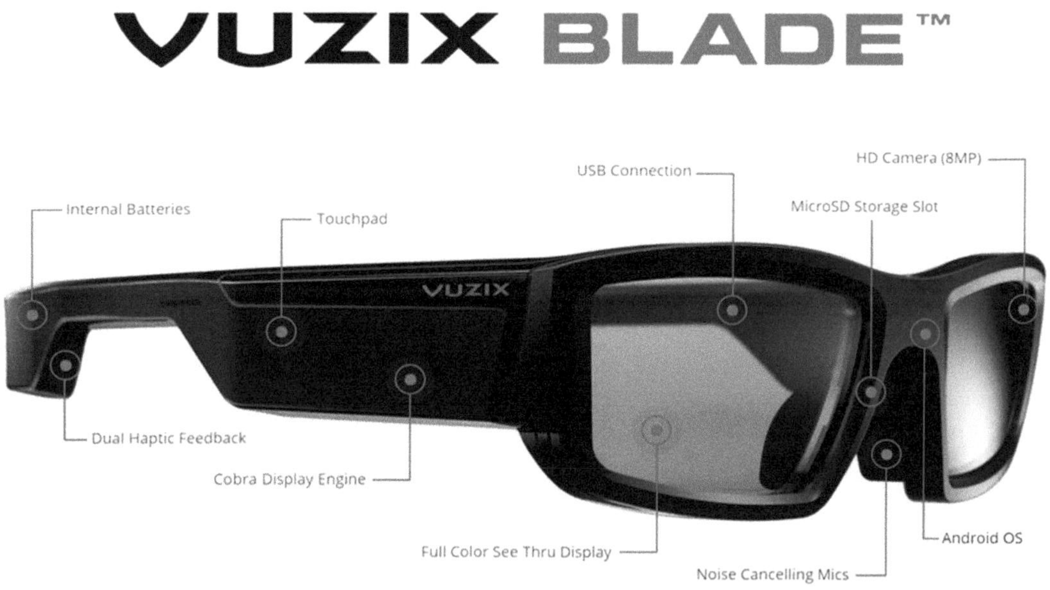

Fig. 5.2 Image of Vuzix Blade (Vuzix Blade® Upgraded Version, 2021)

can augment reality by overlaying pertinent information on top of the user's visual field: projecting a bi-dimensional image on the right lens, the display user interface. Moreover, it can also trigger haptic/vibratory feedback on its right and left temples. Thus, when the Gait Tutor smartphone app sends real-time feedback, the user receives the SG multisensory cues without any action needed.

During the testing protocol, the mGait system was used for gait monitoring and to evaluate spatiotemporal gait parameters, it is a CE-marked medical device from mHealth Technologies (Assessment—mTEST3, mHealth Technologies 2021). The Gait Tutor system used two inertial sensors applied to the feet and transmitted data via Bluetooth to the smartphone app.

Several spatiotemporal gait parameters were considered for the motor evaluation: gait speed, stride length, swing time variability, cadence variability, stance time variability, gait speed variability, stride length variability, cadence, swing time, stance time, cadence asymmetry, swing time asymmetry, stance time asymmetry, and stride length asymmetry (Peterson and Horak 2016). Hence, these parameters were defined as a benchmark to compare the different performances of the trials with users.

The gait rehabilitation solution presented in this book wants to allow therapists to apply tailored rehabilitation programs based on individual patient sensory preferences, cognitive aspects, and medical knowledge.

After several evaluations of commercial SG models responding to the project's technological requirements, the multidisciplinary team finally chose Vuzix Blade SG to submit sensory cues to the users (Fig. 5.2).

This device loads the Android 5.1.1 operating system and weighs 90 gr. It contains many of the capabilities of a standard Android SP in an unobtrusive head-mounted form factor. Blade SG can augment reality by overlaying pertinent information on top of the user's visual field: projecting a bi-dimensional image on the right lens representing the display user interface. Besides, their embedded camera and microphone can capture information about the user environment and handle voice control, while inertial sensors can track the user's head movement. Interestingly, it also can trigger dual haptic/proprioceptive feedback on its right and left temples.

5.4 Creating Phase (C1P3)

The multidisciplinary team developed several design solutions applying UCD principles to evaluate human requirements extrapolated from scientific literature and the interaction with representatives of the selected categories of users.

Signals submitted to the user belonged to three typologies, each one specifically linked to a single sensory channel. The visual stimulus was projected to the user through SG, in the upper left part of the right lens; the acoustic stimulus was provided through traditional wireless earphones; and, finally, the vibratory stimulus was exerted by the temples of SG on the support points. Stimulations occur through cues that do not represent or pronounce the action to be performed but rather try to induce it through simple and intuitive communication, not requiring cognitive or interpretative processing by the user.

The effect of sensory cues aimed at improving gait performances: increasing stride speed and length, and harmonizing the stride phases with the regulatory values from the literature. The author decided to experiment with messages primarily focused on rhythmic transmission that can regulate the cadence of the step on the frequency suggested by the stimuli (100 steps/min) (Imbesi and Corzani 2023).

Visual cues were designed to provide the user with a suggestion on the cadence he should adopt, not providing images not requiring a cognitive interpretation but a rhythmic cadence to follow, without distracting the person from the sight focus of the performing path. Furthermore, it was decided to avoid complex writings and icons, choosing basic images not needing an interpretation. Among the simple analyzed images and shapes, the circle was considered immediate and repurposed in several variations.

The visual signals were developed according to a basic module of two "beats" (intended as right and left steps) played in a loop for the appropriate duration, according to the personal frequency previously set (in the present experiment 100 bpm).

After analyzing different color palettes through the SG display (indoor and outdoor, and different lighting conditions), the selected colors were white and purple in several degrees of saturation because of their visibility in different environmental conditions.

Regarding visualization, the multidisciplinary team defined two possible solutions: two-figure patterns, projected following the right and left steps; and six-figure patterns which should create a sort of graphic animation where the right step corresponds to frame one, and the left step to frame four.

Regarding the number of images and their combination of the projected figures, three compositional solutions were selected as most easy to interpret: the single central figure, the single tilting figure, and the double tilting figure.

The auditive patterns, like the visual ones, aim to influence the users to a predetermined cadence to adapt to their own pace. For the design of the cues belonging to this typology, rhythmic sounds were preferred, because they can be set to annoy the user as little as possible. The rhythms suggested by the metronome, or sounds typical of the world of robotics, have been limited because it was considered that they transmitted feelings of anxiety and burden, preferring those families of sounds closer to the human and musical environments. It was also preferred to exclude the reproduction of a single repetitive sound, more bothering and overwhelming, in favor of some different ones in which melodic attitude suggests a rhythmic alternation in gait guided by a regular combined movement, as evoking the right and left step.

Vibratory cues are exercised by SG on the support points of the right and left temples. Among the three signals, the vibration presented the lower possibility of variation, being monotonic and programmable in the duration variable only.

Vibratory cue variants were developed with the objective of inviting the person to a regular pace of steps. The adopted principle of this design strategy is to provide a rhythm with right and left vibrations corresponding to the impact of the right and left footsteps during the walk.

Developing Design and Technological Solutions

Referring to motor impairments typical of PD, the multidisciplinary team identified several spatiotemporal gait parameters as significant for the motor evaluation as gait speed, stride length, swing time variability, cadence variability, stance time variability, gait speed variability, stride length variability, cadence, swing time, stance time, cadence asymmetry, swing time asymmetry, stance time asymmetry, and stride length asymmetry. These parameters were the benchmarks to compare the different performances obtained during the trials with users.

The novel nature of the mHealth proposed solution is to allow a multisensory approach, where visual and proprioceptive signals complement the auditory feedback. To achieve multisensory stimulation, the Gait Tutor system was integrated with commercial smart glasses for augmented reality applications.

The mHealth system presented in this study was essentially composed of three elements:

- The inertial sensor nodes: two worn on the shoes and one on the trunk;
- An Android Smartphone (SP) app with onboard algorithms able to compute gait features (and generate verbal feedback);
- An Android SG app to generate augmented multisensory feedback (visual and proprioceptive).

Thus, the Gait Tutor system was composed of an SP app processing data streamed from the IMUs positioned on the user's shoes, and it elaborates gait parameters to trigger real-time verbal feedback on gait. Innovatively, the SP app was modified to allow information exchange via Bluetooth with the SG. Thus, when the SP app triggers real-time feedback, the user can receive the SG visual and vibratory cues without any additional action.

Building Prototypes

The designing phase developed many different cues. Some of them, identified as the most effective ones by the multidisciplinary team, were selected to be finally tested with the project users (Imbesi and Corzani 2023).

Specifically, the final cues adopted for the testing process were:

- 6 visual cues (A1:A6)
- 6 auditory cues (B1:B6)
- 2 vibratory cues (C1, C2)
- 2 cues to verify the signal (Z1:Z3)
- 3 multisensory cues (D1:D3)

(A1) It represents a simple pattern using only two images of circles simulating right and left oscillation. It can be defined as a double right-left figure. Beats identified as steps are placed on the first and the second images.

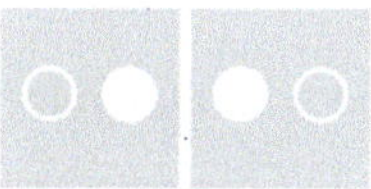

(A2) It represents an animated pattern consisting of six images representing a sort of circular pulse. It can be defined as a central figure flashing. Beats identified as steps are placed on the first and the second images.

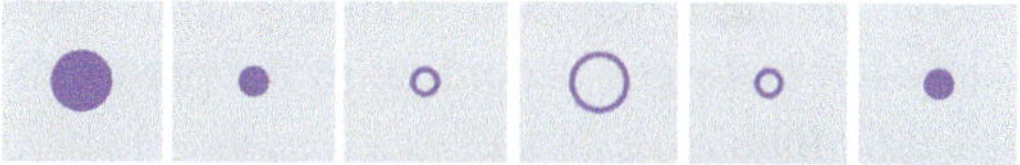

(A3) It represents an animated pattern consisting of 6 images. It can be defined as a central tilting figure. Beats identified as steps are placed on the first and the fourth images.

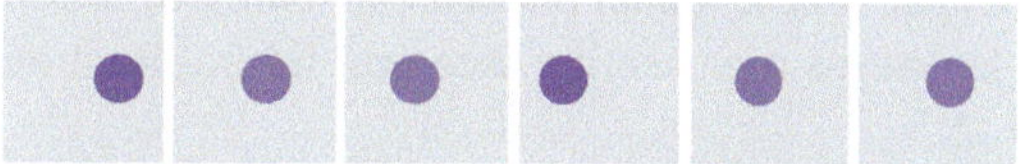

(A4) It represents an animated pattern consisting of 6 images. It can be defined as a central tilting figure. Beats identified as steps are placed on the first and the fourth images.

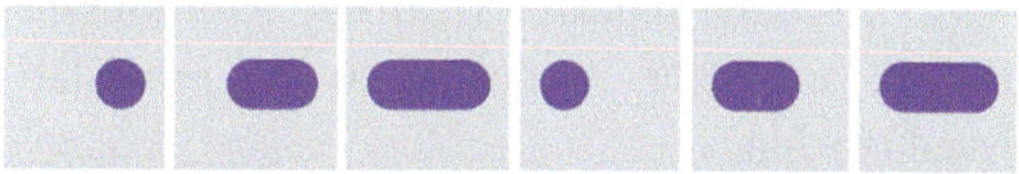

(A5) It represents an animated pattern consisting of 6 images. It can be defined as a double left-right flashing figure. Beats identified as steps are placed on the first and the fourth images.

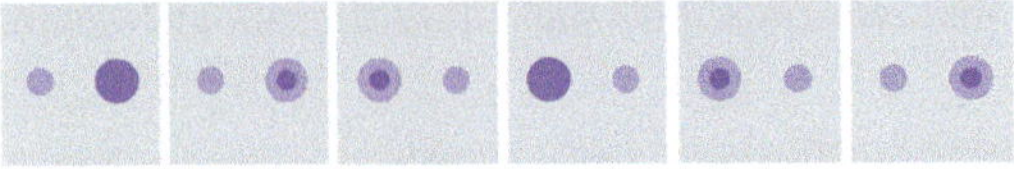

(A6) It represents an animated pattern consisting of 6 images. It can be defined as a double figure tilting right-left, top-bottom. Beats identified as steps are placed on the first and the fourth images.

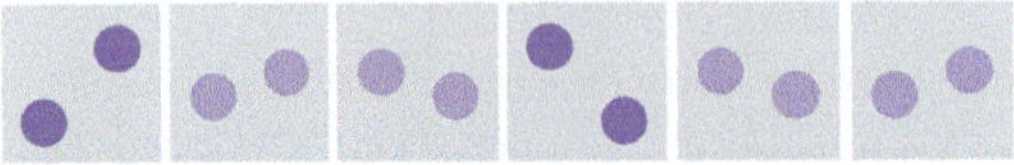

(B1) It consists of a rhythmic sound played by a metronome.
(B2) It consists of a motif performed with two musical instruments (double bass, organ).
(B3) It consists of a motif performed with more musical instruments (double bass, organ, marimba).
(B4) It consists of a motif played with electronic sound (dark).
(B5) It consists of a motif played with electronic sound (ringing).
(B6) It consists of a motif performed with electronic sound (artificial).
(C1) A vibratory pattern consisting of 1 single (short) vibration repeated regularly and alternately left and right, according to the pre-established rhythm.
(C2) Vibratory pattern composed of 2 different vibrations (short-long) reproduced in a regular and alternating way respectively on the right and on the left, according to the pre-established rhythm.
(Z1) A simple visual pattern consisting of 2 single images representing a central figure. Beat on 1, 2.
(Z2) Auditory cue consisting of a motif performed with musical instruments (double bass_marimba).
(Z3) Vibratory pattern made up of 1 single (long) vibration repeated regularly and alternating left and right, according to the pre-established rhythm.
(D1) Visual A5 + auditory B3
(D2) Visual A4 + Vibratory C2
(D3) Visual A3 + Auditory B2 + Vibratory C1

5.5 Verifying Phase (C1P4)

During this last phase of the first design cycle, designed sensory cues were tested with users to collect qualitative and quantitative information that could help the analysis and interpretation of the obtained results.

Qualitative information was obtained thanks to a short questionnaire submitted to each user while testing the cues, while quantitative information was analyzed thanks to gait data monitored during the trial (Imbesi and Corzani 2023).

This information was then elaborated and interpreted to obtain evaluations and users' needs to be used in the final Qualitative Function Deployment (QFD) matrix (Mincolelli et al. 2020) for the simultaneous comparison of factors influencing users' gait in these tests.

Qualitative Information

Qualitative information was primarily obtained from the submission to each user of a questionnaire divided into questions with closed or open answers.

The individual interview was divided into two parts: the first was specific on submitted sensory cues, while the second was on the user's perception of smart glasses.

Questionnaire On Sensory Cues

Was it unpleasant to receive this signal? 1 2 3 4 5
How hard was it to match the pace? 1 2 3 4 5

Open Questionnaire On Smart Glasses

How do you feel wearing smart glasses?
What do you think about it aesthetically?
Is there something that makes you uncomfortable?

How long do you think you can wear smart glasses?
In what contexts could you imagine using them?
How do you think your walk has changed after the stimuli received?

Quantitative Information

Concerning the quantitative data collection, a testing protocol was applied to monitor several gait parameters about users' performances.

Operators collected users' data such as age, height, sex, and dominant foot, to understand the characteristics of the performances of the different involved people.

Everything was filmed to have a gold standard for doubts (frame both the walking subject and the operator sending the stimulus).

During the tests, operators equipped every user with the mGait system and sent them the selected sensory cues via an ad-hoc smartphone app (Fig. 5.3).

It is relevant to point out that in this experiment, all the cues were set on the cadence of 100 steps per minute, a value close to the average walking rhythm suggested by the literature (Rochester et al. 2010).

At the beginning of the set procedure, before carrying out the tests with sensory cues, a walk was performed along the same path but without the induction of Z signals to take the parameters related to this test as a reference concerning the following ones.

The user was then invited to perform the path using his usual pace, and between 5 and 7 m from the start of the walk (range granted depending on the basic step length of the tested user, so the tests of different users can be comparable in duration and the number of steps), the cue was transmitted. It was then interrupted only at the end of the path (the subject usually walks at least 15 m after receiving the signal).

Regarding the submission of the stimulation, attention was dedicated to the correct synchronization between the incoming signal and the user's cadence of the walk: the signal was then sent to the subject while the right heel touched the floor, and the step was accomplished (Fig. 5.4).

To verify the perceptual impact of the monosensory stimuli with the least possible conditioning, operators carried out the first three tests without providing information to users either on the type of signal that was going to be received or on the behavior that the person was supposed to adopt.

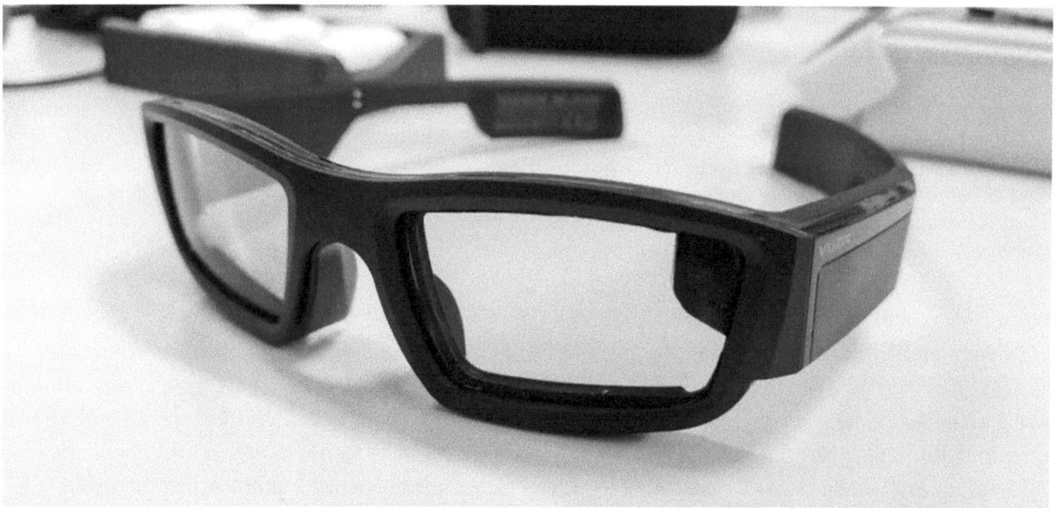

Fig. 5.3 Users' equipment during the testing protocol

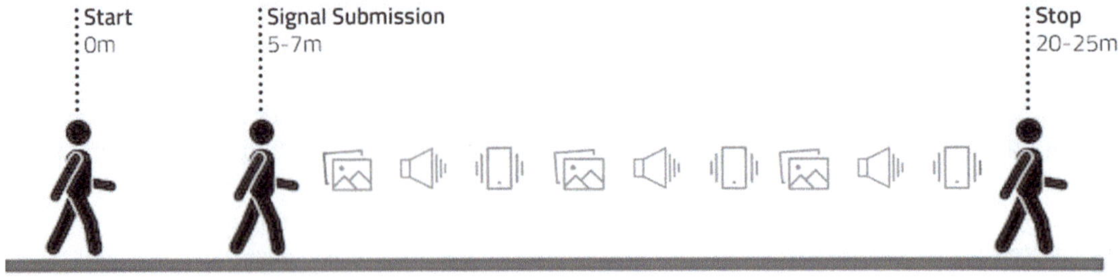

Fig. 5.4 Representation of the path conceived for the users' testing.

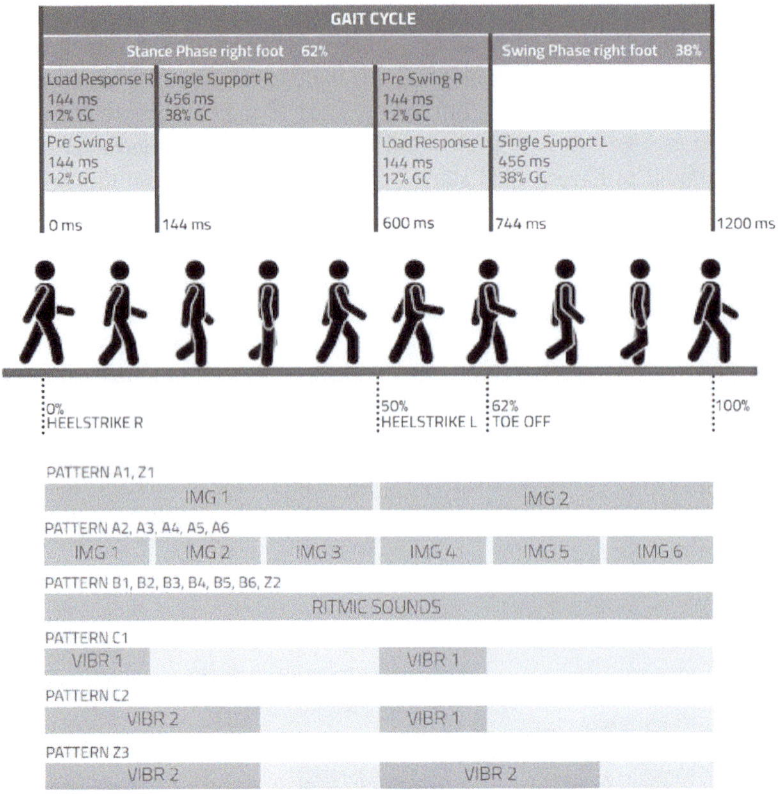

Fig. 5.5 Representation of a gait cycle and indication of the different phases and their duration. In the lower part of the diagram, the individual signals are submitted according to their temporal distribution associated with the phases of the step. The durations were calculated according to the given cadence of 100 steps per minute (Iosa et al. 2013)

Subsequently, during the second part of the test, the user was invited to align with the cadence suggested by the mono or multi-sensory submitted stimulus (Iosa et al. 2013) (Fig. 5.5).

In total, each subject will perform 21 tests following this scheme:

1 baseline trial without cues as the reference;

3 monosensory trials with randomized administration order (Z1, Z2, Z3);

14 monosensory tests and 3 multisensory tests with randomized administration order (A1: A6, B1: B6, C1: C2, D1: D3).

5.6 Conclusions

The first design cycle of the PASSO research project aimed to design and test several prototypes of sensory cues for the training of the gait of patients affected by PD. The identified primary users were PD patients, and the secondary ones were medical and technical operators. Several sensory cues were designed, the auditory ones submitted by earphones, the visual ones by SG, and the vibratory ones by the SG's lenses; even some multisensory cues were developed. The cues prototypes were used in a testing protocol where users had to walk along a path receiving sensory signals suggesting a cadence to align to.

The applied UCD approach allowed the involvement of users in the definition of the most effective sensory signals, improving the potential usability of the system. Moreover, the used methodology considered each design element of the project as a single cycle of the design process, and divided each cycle into the phases of planning, analyzing, creating, and verifying, giving a structured process to the entire project.

References

"Assessment—mTEST3," mHealth Technologies. Accessed Nov 08 2021. [Online]. Available: http://mhealthtechnologies.it/products-wearable-sensors-smartphone-apps/assessment-mtest3/

J.C. Ayena, L.E. Tremblay, M.J.-D. Otis, B.-A.J. Ménélas, Comparing auditory, visual and vibrotactile cues in individuals with Parkinson's disease for reducing risk of falling over different types of soil. Somatosens. Mot. Res. **34**(4), 226–234 (2017). https://doi.org/10.1080/08990220.2017.1421157

M. Capecci et al., Postural rehabilitation and kinesio taping for axial postural disorders in Parkinson's disease. Arch. Phys. Med. Rehabil. **95**(6), 1067–1075 (2014). https://doi.org/10.1016/j.apmr.2014.01.020

F. Casamassima, A. Ferrari, B. Milosevic, P. Ginis, E. Farella, L. Rocchi, A wearable system for gait training in subjects with Parkinson's disease. Sensors **14**(4), Art. no. 4 (2014). https://doi.org/10.3390/s140406229

S. Davidsdottir, A. Cronin-Golomb, A. Lee, Visual and spatial symptoms in Parkinson's disease. Vision. Res. **45**(10), 1285–1296 (2005). https://doi.org/10.1016/j.visres.2004.11.006

C.A. Davie, A review of Parkinson's disease. Br. Med. Bull. **86**(1), 109–127 (2008). https://doi.org/10.1093/bmb/ldn013

D. Ferrazzoli, P. Ortelli, G. Madeo, N. Giladi, G.M. Petzinger, G. Frazzitta, Basal ganglia and beyond: the interplay between motor and cognitive aspects in Parkinson's disease rehabilitation. Neurosci. Biobehav. Rev. **90**, 294–308 (2018). https://doi.org/10.1016/j.neubiorev.2018.05.007

H.R. Gonçalves, A.M. Rodrigues, C.P. Santos, Vibrotactile biofeedback devices in Parkinson's disease: a narrative review. Med. Biol. Eng. Comput. **59**(6), 1185–1199 (2021). https://doi.org/10.1007/s11517-021-02365-3

V.A. Goodwin, S.H. Richards, R.S. Taylor, A.H. Taylor, J.L. Campbell, The effectiveness of exercise interventions for people with Parkinson's disease: a systematic review and meta-analysis. Mov. Disord. off. J. Mov. Disord. Soc. **23**(5), 631–640 (2008). https://doi.org/10.1002/mds.21922

S. Imbesi, M. Corzani, Multisensory cues for gait rehabilitation with smart glasses: methodology, design, and results of a preliminary pilot. Sensors **23**(2), Art. no. 2 (2023). https://doi.org/10.3390/s23020874

M. Iosa et al., The golden ratio of gait harmony: repetitive proportions of repetitive gait phases. BioMed Res. Int. **2013**, 918642 (2013). https://doi.org/10.1155/2013/918642

I. Lim et al., Effects of external rhythmical cueing on gait in patients with Parkinson's disease: a systematic review. Clin. Rehabil. **19**(7), 695–713 (2005). https://doi.org/10.1191/0269215505cr906oa

G. Mincolelli, S. Imbesi, M. Zallio, Collaborative quality function deployment. A methodology for enabling co-design research practice, in *Advances in Design for Inclusion*, ed. by G. Di Bucchianico, in Advances in Intelligent Systems and Computing (Cham: Springer International Publishing, 2020), pp. 91–99. https://doi.org/10.1007/978-3-030-20444-0_9

A. Nieuwboer, R. Dom, W. De Weerdt, K. Desloovere, S. Fieuws, E. Broens-Kaucsik, Abnormalities of the spatiotemporal characteristics of gait at the onset of freezing in Parkinson's disease. Mov. Disord. **16**(6), 1066–1075 (2001). https://doi.org/10.1002/mds.1206

A. Nieuwboer et al., Cueing training in the home improves gait-related mobility in Parkinson's disease: the RESCUE trial. J. Neurol. Neurosurg. Psychiatry **78**(2), 134–140 (2007). https://doi.org/10.1136/jnnp.200X.097923

D.S. Peterson, F.B. Horak, Neural control of walking in people with parkinsonism. Physiol. Bethesda Md. **31**(2), 95–107 (2016). https://doi.org/10.1152/physiol.00034.2015

D.S. Peterson, K. Smulders, Cues and attention in parkinsonian gait: potential mechanisms and future directions. Front. Neurol. **6**, 255 (2015). https://doi.org/10.3389/fneur.2015.00255

G.M. Petzinger, B.E. Fisher, S. McEwen, J.A. Beeler, J.P. Walsh, M.W. Jakowec, Exercise-enhanced neuroplasticity targeting motor and cognitive circuitry in Parkinson's disease. Lancet Neurol. **12**(7), 716–726 (2013). https://doi.org/10.1016/S1474-4422(13)70123-6

P.A. Rocha, G.M. Porfírio, H.B. Ferraz, V.F.M. Trevisani, Effects of external cues on gait parameters of Parkinson's disease patients: a systematic review. Clin. Neurol. Neurosurg. **124**, 127–134 (2014). https://doi.org/10.1016/j.clineuro.2014.06.026

L. Rochester et al., Evidence for motor learning in Parkinson's disease: acquisition, automaticity and retention of cued gait performance after training with external rhythmical cues. Brain Res. **1319**, 103–111 (2010). https://doi.org/10.1016/j.brainres.2010.01.001

T.C. Rubinstein, N. Giladi, J.M. Hausdorff, The power of cueing to circumvent dopamine deficits: a review of physical therapy treatment of gait disturbances in Parkinson's disease. Mov. Disord. off. J. Mov. Disord. Soc. **17**(6), 1148–1160 (2002). https://doi.org/10.1002/mds.10259

Á. Sánchez-Ferro, W. Maetzler, Advances in sensor and wearable technologies for Parkinson's disease. Mov. Disord. off. J. Mov. Disord. Soc. **31**(9), 1257 (2016). https://doi.org/10.1002/mds.26746

L. Shams, A.R. Seitz, Benefits of multisensory learning. Trends Cogn. Sci. **12**(11), 411–417 (2008). https://doi.org/10.1016/j.tics.2008.07.006

S.J. Spaulding, B. Barber, M. Colby, B. Cormack, T. Mick, M.E. Jenkins, Cueing and gait improvement among people with Parkinson's disease: a meta-analysis. Arch. Phys. Med. Rehabil. **94**(3), 562–570 (2013). https://doi.org/10.1016/j.apmr.2012.10.026

C.L. Tomlinson et al., Physiotherapy intervention in Parkinson's disease: systematic review and meta-analysis. BMJ **345**, e5004 (2012). https://doi.org/10.1136/bmj.e5004

T.-H. Tsai, W.-Y. Lin, Y.-S. Chang, P.-C. Chang, M.-Y. Lee, Technology anxiety and resistance to change behavioral study of a wearable cardiac warming system using an extended TAM for older adults. PLoS ONE **15**(1), e0227270 (2020). https://doi.org/10.1371/journal.pone.0227270

"User-Centered Design Process Map." Accessed Sep 19 2023. [Online]. Available: https://www.usability.gov/how-to-and-tools/resources/ucd-map.html

"Vuzix Blade® Upgraded Version." Accessed Nov 08 2021. [Online]. Available: https://www.vuzix.com/products/blade-smart-glasses-upgraded

E.E.H. van Wegen, M.A. Hirsch, M. Huiskamp, G. Kwakkel, Harnessing cueing training for neuroplasticity in Parkinson disease. Top. Geriatr. Rehabil. **30**(1), 46–57 (2014). https://doi.org/10.1097/TGR.0000000000000005

B.K. Wiederhold, Time to port augmented reality health apps to smart glasses? Cyberpsychology Behav. Soc. Netw. **16**(3), 157–158 (2013). https://doi.org/10.1089/cyber.2013.1503

6 Cycle 1: Interpretation of Results

Abstract

This chapter, describes results gained during the first design cycle of the PASSO research project, regarding the design of smart sensory cues submitting images, sounds, and vibrations to the users affected by Parkinson's disease to influence their gait. The testing protocol described in the previous chapter involved several users and allowed the mHealth system to collect data about the gait of tested people, visualize results, and share outcomes with the multidisciplinary team to make considerations from different research fields. In the second part of the cycle, the author describes a novel application of the Quality Function Deployment as a tool to combine the results obtained by the tested sensory cues, towards a classification of the most effective ones.

6.1 Testing with Users

This chapter follows the previous one, describing the methodological process of the first design cycle of the research project PASSO, developing a system providing sensory cues to rehabilitate the gait and posture of people affected by Parkinson's disease (PD).

In the following part, the author analyzes and suggests an interpretation of the results obtained during the testing phase of the first cycle of the project (Imbesi and Mincolelli 2022).

Moreover, results are represented in graphical schemes aiming to provide a quick and easy lecture to each member of the multidisciplinary team, independently from the scientific background, to encourage a shared discussion about collected users' data (Imbesi and Corzani 2023).

In this design cycle, it was chosen to involve test users not belonging to a specific category reporting health diseases. The main reason was that, from the pandemic perspective, it was chosen not to expose frailty people to potential health risks. Another reason is that in this first part of the experimentation, it was possible to consider a Human-Centered approach considering the human perception instead of PD people's.

The following sections describe the outputs of the single interviews submitted to every volunteer participating in the testing protocol. The discussed arguments were Smart Glasses (SG) and the sensory cues.

User 1 (U1):

U1 usually wears glasses but feels SG is heavier than his ones. He appreciates SG's aspect. He has no problems in perceiving and reading images. He thinks he could wear SG all day long, at the same time he wears his daily glasses. He would wear SG on his own instead of a smartwatch.

S. Imbesi, *Inclusive Design of a Smart Device for People with Parkinson's Disease*, Design For Inclusion 4, https://doi.org/10.1007/978-3-031-58249-3_6

Regarding the testing protocol, he thinks cues changed his way of walking. He had some problems with a specific auditory signal because he could not find the rhythm to follow. He thinks the easiest cues were the vibratory ones than the visual ones, and the most difficult were the auditory ones apart from the metronome. He didn't like that SG images were projected in the center of the lens, and he would have preferred to see images on the sides of his field of view. He thinks vibration is the less enjoyable signal but the easiest to follow, and the other ones are neither enjoyable nor annoying.

User 2 (U2):

U2 usually doesn't wear glasses. Initially, he felt SG a little heavy, but when he concentrated on the path he forgot he was wearing them. Aesthetically he thinks SG is heavy due to the thick frame. Regarding the projection, sometimes he felt quite disoriented and alarmed by the perception of light and images when he wasn't aware they were coming. He would wear SG for a maximum of a few hours, not more. He would wear SG for sports or daily activities such as searching a map while cycling.

He didn't know if his walk changed with cues during the testing protocol, but he thought it was more rhythmic. In his opinion, the auditory and vibratory signals were more effective, and the auditory was the most relaxing and not demanding of the user's attention. Visual signals were more difficult due to this feeling of alertness. He thinks multi-sensory cues were pretty annoying and demanded too much attention. The more acceptable stimuli for him was the multisensory one matching audio and vibration.

User 3 (U3):

U3 usually doesn't wear glasses, she perceived SG as annoying because they were too heavy. She would wear them for the shortest possible time. She wouldn't wear SG in her daily life, maybe for sports.

She thinks that during tests she was able to follow the suggested rhythm. She perceived the easiest cues as the auditory and vibratory, while images were confusing. She thinks the metronome was the easiest to follow, but it transmitted some anxiety. She felt balance problems with visual cues.

User 4 (U4):

U4 usually doesn't wear glasses, but he did not feel SG was uncomfortable. He thinks he would wear SG for a maximum of 4–5 h. He would use SG for running training or similar functions but doesn't know if it is possible.

Regarding the testing phase, he doesn't know if he could be uniform to the suggested rhythm. While receiving submitted cues, he thought they suggested different cadences because he perceived non-uniform sensations of cues urgency. He perceived images as very slow and vibrations as very quick, as they were not aligned, but indeed they suggested the same rhythm.

User 5 (U5):

U5 usually doesn't wear glasses, but he felt SG's temples tight on his head. He would wear SG for 1 h, not more. He could preferably use SG if they consent to a perspective projection and recognition of elements in the environment.

During the testing protocol, he perceived vibration as a stopping, like he did something wrong. Auditory cues were his favorite, while he did not like visual cues. He thinks his gait changed after signals but couldn't describe how.

6.2 Qualitative and Quantitative Evaluations

During the testing protocol, the multidisciplinary team collected information and data about users' performances while receiving sensory cues. These data were divided into qualitative information expressed by users reporting their feelings and sensations about the testing protocols, and quantitative data from wearable sensors collecting users' spatiotemporal gait parameters.

Thanks to visual instruments and strategies, the following figures allowed significant considerations about data collected during the testing protocol (Imbesi and Mincolelli 2022; Imbesi and Corzani 2023). The quick reading and easy interpretation of complex tables of numbers considerably helped the working team members without technical knowledge in this field to get and understand more information about the ongoing project, enhancing their contribution to the whole design process.

The collection of this information allowed researchers to extrapolate the users' needs to be used in the final evaluation elaborated with the help of the Quality Function Deployment tool (QFD) (Mincolelli et al. 2020a).

Qualitative Tests' Outcomes

Starting from answers given by users during the individual interviews, the multidisciplinary team analyzed perceptions about users' perceived difficulty in following the cue to evaluate the cues' effectiveness and usability.

In this section are reported evaluations of qualitative information given by users about feelings and perceptions during the testing protocol.

It investigated the following aspects of submitted cues:

- perceived invasivity and annoyance;
- perceived difficulty in following the signal.

Cues' Perceived Invasivity and Annoyance

After each test, users answered the question: "How invasive and annoying was this cue?" (Fig. 6.1). Tested people assigned every feedback a mark from 1 to 5 (1 not invasive, 5 very invasive).

From the representation in Fig. 6.1, it is possible to notice that visual cues were the most annoying for most people, auditory cues were less disturbing depending on the sounds, and vibratory cues were perceived halfway between the previous ones. Multi-sensory cues were perceived as very annoying due to the amount of involved sensories.

The multidisciplinary team analyzed even the variance of users' answers to understand if

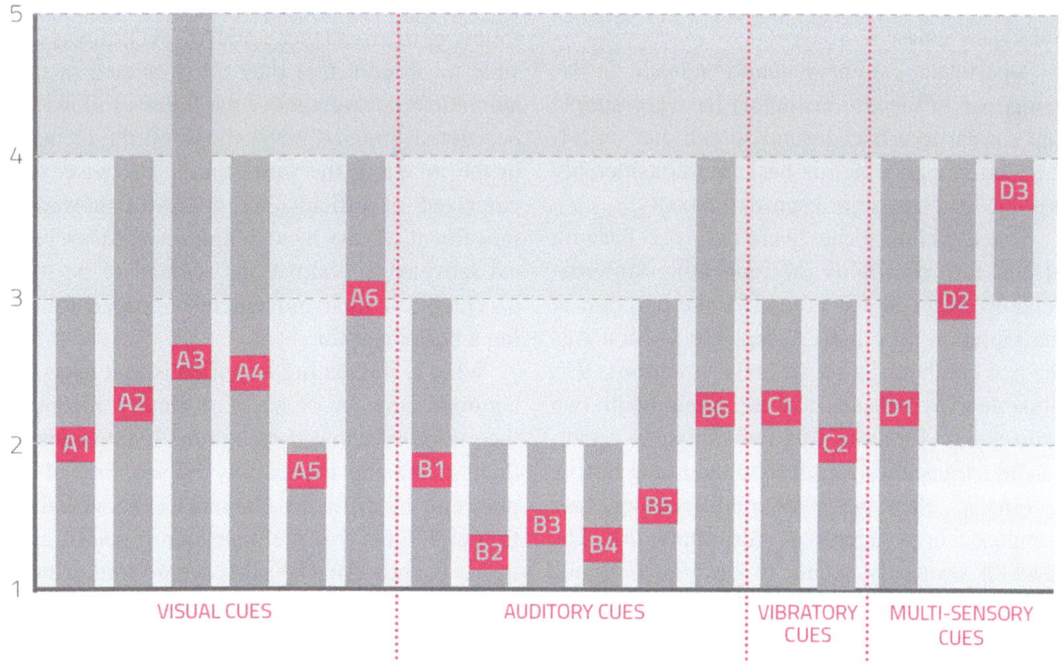

Fig. 6.1 Graphical representation of users' answers on how invasive and annoying the cues were

they all perceived cues as invasive and annoying in the same way. From Fig. 6.1 it is possible to notice that some cues, especially auditive ones, are similarly perceived in all tests (A1, A5, B1, B2, B3, B4, B5, C1, C2, D2, D3); for some others, particularly for visual cues, the users' scores are both low and high (A2, A3, A4, A6, B6, D1), highlighting the influence of personal preferences and attitudes in the perception of invasivity.

It is interesting to observe that the most disturbing visual cues (A6, A3, A4) were the ones not presenting a fixed point for anchoring the view; conversely, the less three annoying ones (A2, A1, A5) present images modifying their color or dimension but not their position. The movement of the circular figure seems to be accepted just if accompanied by a fixed point where the user can anchor his view to find balance and stability.

Regarding auditory cues, the image reveals that the more the cue is composed of electronic and artificial sounds, the more it is perceived as invasive and annoying (B6, B1, B5); otherwise, it is less disturbing when played by a few musical instruments (B3, B4, B2), that seem to be a more familiar and relaxing condition in the users' perception.

A particular comment should be made on B4, composed of electronic sounds but very simple and similar to a background sound; and on B1, the metronome, which is basic but considerably artificial and transmits a sense of anxiety.

Tested vibratory cues were only two because of the low possibility of replicating different versions of the signal except for the duration of the vibration. The most acceptable version was the one combining two different vibrations. It is possible to hypothesize that the version with two short equal vibrations was too similar to a metronome, transmitting a sense of incoming hurry.

Finally, users perceived multi-sensory cues composed of 3 signals as very annoying. The level of invasivity seems to be related to the number of involved senses and the complexity of the signal. Considering multi-sensory cues composed of 2 signals, the less disturbing was the one comprising the visual and auditory cues.

Cues' Perceived Difficulty in Following the Signal

After the testing phase, participants answered the question "How difficult was it to follow the rhythm suggested by this cue?". Then they gave each cue from 1 to 5 points (1 not invasive, 5 very invasive) (Fig. 6.2).

Figure 6.2 shows that visual cues and several auditory signals were the most challenging to adapt to; the other visual cues, with the vibratory and multisensory ones, were considered moderately difficult to follow. The metronome auditory signal was the only one perceived as moderately difficult by the tested people.

The figure also considers the variance of answers to observe if all users felt the cues as difficult to follow in the same way. It is possible to notice that only some visual and auditory signals were similarly perceived in each trial (A1, A2, A5, B1, B2, B3, D2); the other ones reported some differences in assigned scores (A3, A4, A6, B4, B5, B6, C1, C2, D1, D3), underlining the significant effect of personal attitudes in the perception of the difficulty of following the suggested rhythm.

Trying to find some common characteristics in visual cues perceived as not too difficult to follow in their cadence (A5, A4, A1), it was possible to observe that they all presented in their animation a movement of the figures following a horizontal line and never move all the elements in the image at the same time; otherwise, cues perceived as difficult (A2, A3, A6), showed no movement, or no fixed points in shift or vertical movement. Animations seemed to be more acceptable if their movement happened following a horizontal line.

What is interesting to notice is that users put auditory cues in order of difficulty following the same order that used authors listing cues for their increasing complexity of sounds and the presence of artificial elements. The visualization highlights that melodies composed of electronic sounds (B6, B5, B4) were more difficult to follow; differently, melodies composed by musical instruments B3, B2, and B4) seemed to be perceived as more effective in suggesting a rhythm.

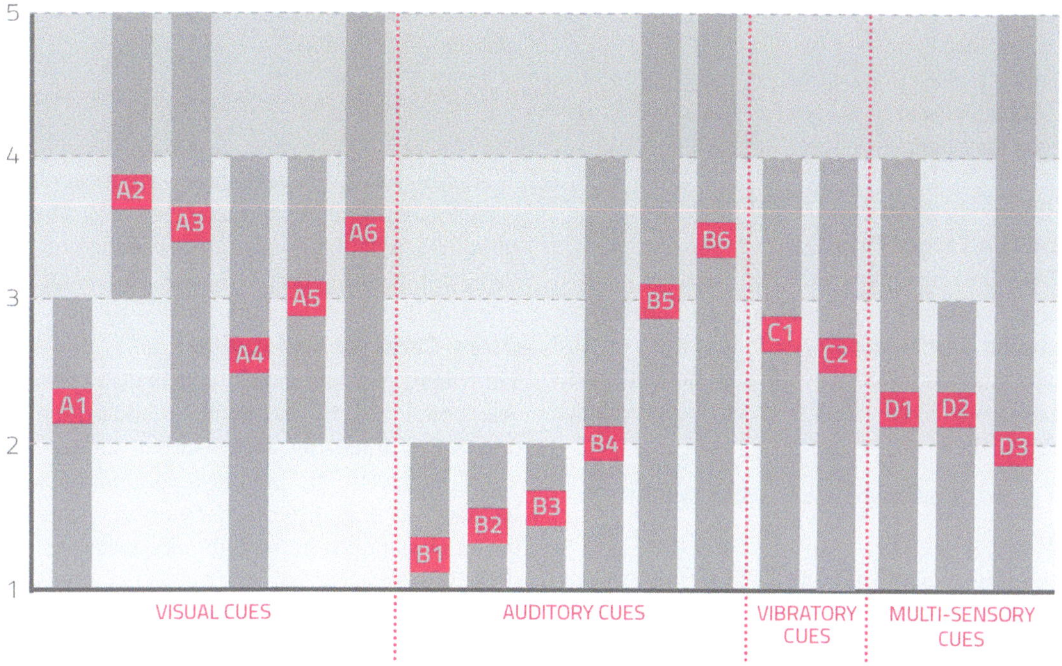

Fig. 6.2 Graphical representation of users' answers on how difficult it was to follow the rhythm suggested by each cue

A special comment should be made on the metronome B1, which was an artificial and simple sound, therefore its effectiveness in giving a rhythm was obvious.

Tested vibratory cues were only two, because of the low possibility of replicating different versions of the signal except for the duration of the vibration. Users perceived the one composed of two short vibrations as less difficult to follow, maybe because its concept is very similar to the metronome one.

Multi-sensory cues using three different senses were perceived as the easiest to follow, it seemed to be related to the number of involved senses and to the redundancy of the signal in suggesting a rhythm. Considering multisensory cues composed of 2 signals, they are perceived as moderately difficult, preferring the one combining visual and auditory cues.

Quantitative Tests' Outcomes

The multidisciplinary team collected several spatiotemporal parameters regarding the users' gait that were elaborated to deduce useful information for the evaluation of the effectiveness of the submitted cues and to plan efficiently the next trial (Imbesi and Corzani 2023).

Parameters considered during this testing protocol were:

- Difference between the user's cadence and the target one;
- Number of steps to reach the cadence of 100 steps/min;
- Users' cadence variability;
- Rhythmic asymmetry: users' asymmetry index on cadence;
- Spatial asymmetry: users' asymmetry index on stride length;

- Stride length;
- Gait speed;
- Swing phase;
- Stance phase;
- Swing phase.

Difference Between Users' Cadence and the Target One

The following figure analyzed cadence median values obtained by making the difference between users' cadence and the target of 100 steps/min. The analysis of this parameter aimed to evaluate the deviation from the target cadence (Fig. 6.3).

$$\Delta Cad = abs\,(Cad - Cadtarget)$$

Auditory and Vibratory cues were most performing because they were the closest to the target cadence of 100 steps/min and with the lowest interquartile range, particularly for B1, B2, B6, C2.

Number of Steps to Reach the Cadence of 100 Steps/Min

This visualization represented the number of steps needed to lead the users' cadence within a value of 95–105 steps/min (5% of the target cadence) for at least 5 steps. If there was no alignment in the trial, the technical operator reported the number of 30 steps, coherent with the steps maximum number, taken after the cue submission (Fig. 6.4).

$$StepTreact = (Cad >= 95\ \&\ Cad <= 105)\ \text{at least 5 steps}$$

Auditory and Vibratory cues were most effective considering this parameter, showing to ease an agile adaptation to the target cadence of 100 steps/min in particular for B4, B5, B6, and C2.

Users' Cadence Variability

The analysis of users' cadence variability was conducted by extracting standard deviation and normalizing the resulting data among tested subjects. The obtained parameters were intended as the difference from the standard deviation obtained in the reference measurement (Fig. 6.5).

$$Cadstd = 1N - 1k = 1NCadk - Cad2$$

Cad: Average Cadence.

N: Number of steps

$$\mathbf{\Delta Cadstd = Cadstd - CadstdREF}$$

Auditory and vibratory signals suggested a more constant and balanced walk than the visual cues, it was possible to observe that their standard deviation was lower than the one registered during the reference session.

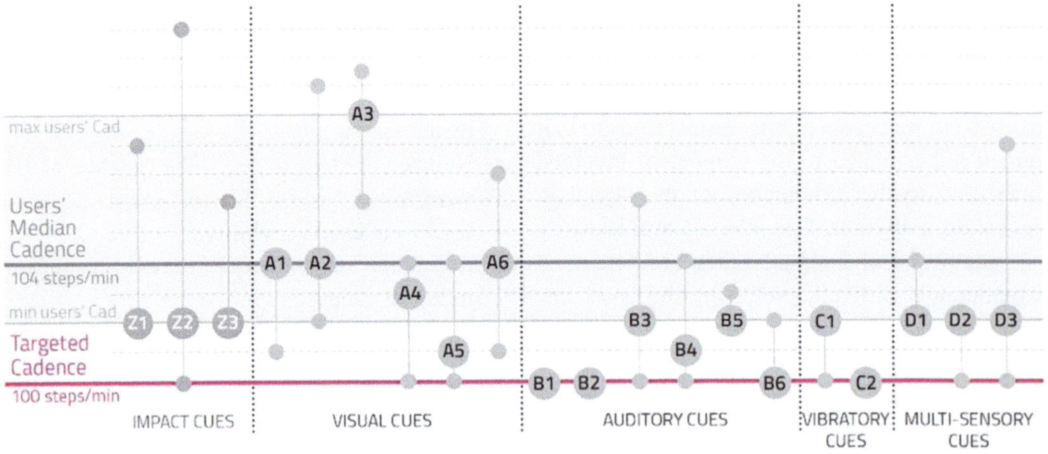

Fig. 6.3 Graphical representation of the users' cadence during each signal

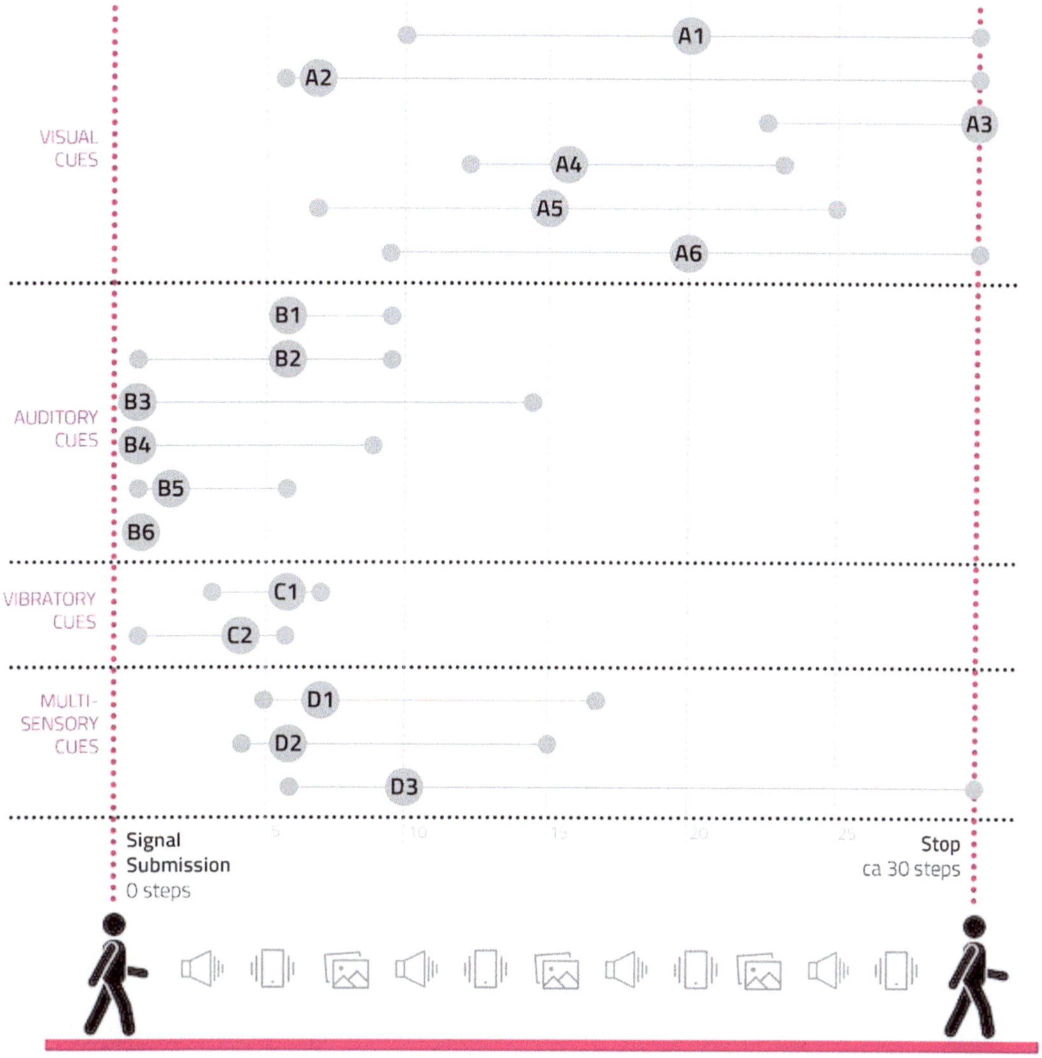

Fig. 6.4 Graphical representation of the number of steps it took for the user to align to the signal

Rhythmic Asymmetry: Users' Asymmetry Index on Cadence

The following figure represents the percentage variation between the average right and left cadence during the performance. Obtained data were normalized among users reporting values as the difference from the cadence asymmetry index gained in the reference trial (Fig. 6.6).

$$\text{CadAsym} = \text{absCadRight} - \text{CadLeft}0.5 * [\text{CadRight} + \text{CadLeft}] * 100$$

Cad: Average Cadence

$$\Delta\textbf{CadAsym} = \textbf{CadAsym} - \textbf{CadAsym REF}$$

This parameter did not lead to a clear interpretation of cues' performances because of the high level of variability of data among analyzed users using the different sensory channels.

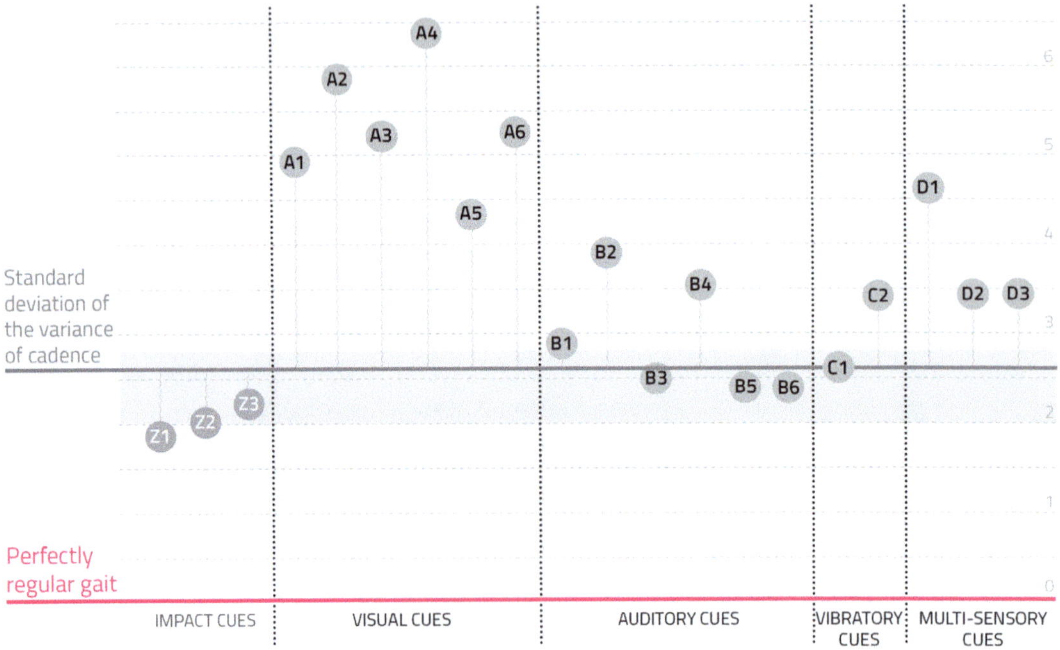

Fig. 6.5 Graphical representation of users' cadence variability

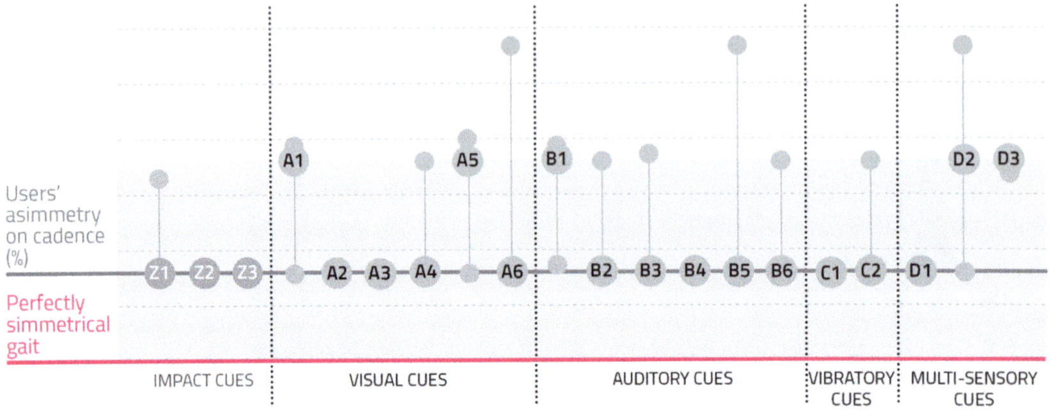

Fig. 6.6 Graphical representation of users' asymmetry in right and left cadence variability

Spatial Asymmetry: Users' Asymmetry Index on Stride Length

This value expresses the percentage of variation between the average right and left stride length measured during the testing protocol. Collected data were normalized among tested subjects, and values were defined as the difference between the stride length asymmetry index, and the one concerning the reference test (Fig. 6.7).

$$\mathrm{SLAsym} = \mathrm{absSLRight} - \mathrm{SLLeft}0.5 * [\mathrm{SLRight} + \mathrm{SLLeft}] * 100$$

SL: Average Stride Length

$$\mathbf{\Delta SLAsym = SLAsym \;\; - SLAsym\ REF}$$

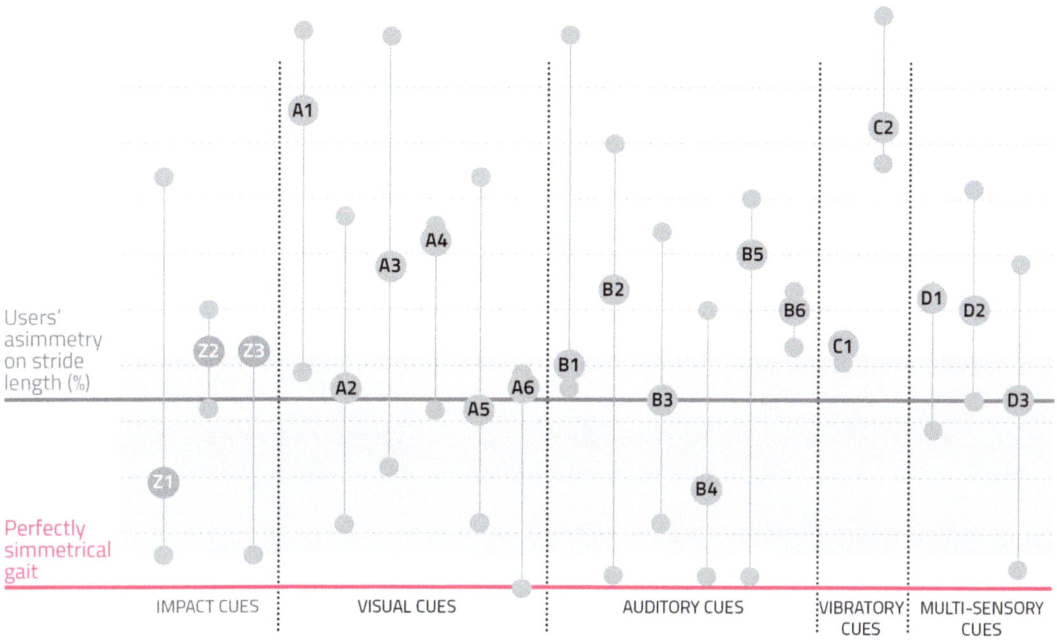

Fig. 6.7 Graphical representation of users' asymmetry in right and left stride length

Figure 6.7 shows a high level of asymmetry in the subjects' stride length, a possible interpretation of this behavior was that users attempted to change their way of walking do adapt to the rhythm suggested by submitted sensory cues.

Other Gait Parameters Describing Results of the Trial

In this section are reported spatiotemporal gait parameters detected in the tests but not used to evaluate cues. These parameters suggest a downgrade of their motor performance following the feedback. This happened probably because the cadence target was generally lower than the user's one, and secondly, because cues can lead to hesitation. Therefore, operators observed a reduction in stride length, gait speed, and swing time, with an increase in stance time.

All reported parameters were related to specific aspects of gait impairments brought by PD disease (Peterson and Horak 2016) (Fig. 6.8).

Graphical Comparisons

Aiming to collect as much information as possible from the experimented tested protocol, the multidisciplinary team decided to make further comparisons on qualitative and quantitative collected feedback (Imbesi and Mincolelli 2022).

Comparison Between Qualitative Feedback

The following figure represents users' answers about their perception of submitted cues, including both the annoyance of the signal and the difficulty in following it (Fig. 6.9).

Looking at Fig. 6.9, visual cues were arduous to follow for users due to the involvement of the visual channel, simultaneously engaged in the walking action. They were even quite invasive and annoying for the same reason.

Auditory cues were more difficult to follow than invasive and annoying, but their overall

DOMAINS OF CONTINUOS GAIT DISTURBANCES	RELATED GAIT ASPECTS	INVOLVED SPATIO-TEMPORAL PARAMETERS
GAIT SLOWNESS	**PACE**	Gait Speed Stride Lenght Swing Time Variability
	RHYTHM	Cadence Swing Time Stance Time
INCREASED VARIABILITY AND ASYMMETRY	**VARIABILITY**	Cadence Variability Stance Time Variability Gait Speed Variability Stride Lenght Variability
	ASYMMETRY	Cadence Asymmetry Swing Time Asymmetry Stance Time Asymmetry
POOR POSTURAL CONTROL	**POSTURAL CONTROL**	Stride Lenght Asymmetry

Fig. 6.8 Domains of PD gait disturbances and related spatio-temporal parameters

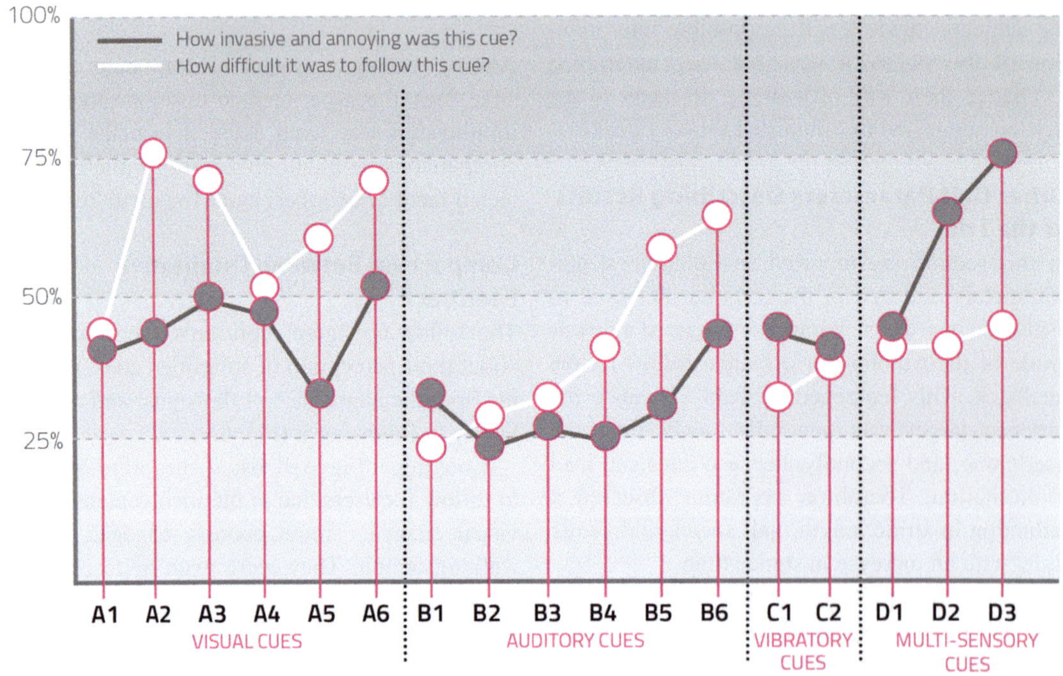

Fig. 6.9 Comparison between answers given by users about single cues' invasiveness and annoyance, and the difficulty in following the signal

perception was the more effective between the different typologies of signals.

Vibratory cues were more invasive and annoying than arduous to follow but with a good perception.

Multisensory cues had the highest degree of invasiveness and annoyance and were slightly difficult to follow. This result could be attributed to the contemporary involvement of two or three sensory channels. The D3 cue engaging all three tested senses, was the one inspiring the worst feelings.

It is interesting to notice that users were able to distinguish different feelings about the signals: in cues A2, A5, B5, and D3, there was a considerable difference between the scores given in the two answers, while differently, for cues A1, A4, C2, D1 most of the users gave almost the same scoring.

Comparison Between Quantitative Feedback

In this section are reported radar schemes that represent users' performances during the submission of visual, auditory, vibratory, and multisensory cues.

Moreover, among quantitative results, a more in-depth evaluation is reported to analyze the variations of the five independent domains peculiar to Parkinsonian gait: pace, rhythm, variability, asymmetry, and postural control (Peterson and Horak 2016).

The author adopted radar plots to assess this analysis during the submission of cues. Thus, within each radar plot, the following outcomes were reported: gait speed, stride length, and swing time variation to evaluate the pace domain; cadence variability, stance time variability, gait speed variability, and stride length variability to evaluate the variability domain; cadence, swing time and stance time to evaluate the rhythm domain; cadence asymmetry, swing time asymmetry, and stance time asymmetry to evaluate the asymmetry domain; and, finally, stride length asymmetry to evaluate the postural control domain.

Collected data were analyzed and reported as a percentage of the baseline trial (reported with 0%). To improve comprehension, for each outcome, we consider a positive effect if the percentage is higher than the reference (0%) (Figs. 6.10, 6.11, 6.12 and 6.13).

Final Needs and Quality Function Deployment

At this point of the design process, the amount of collected information, parameters, and considerations was arduous to manage to obtain an accurate hierarchization of the cue's effectiveness. Therefore, the Quality Function Deployment (QFD) was used to manage the complexity of collected data and judge the functionality and usability of every cue, in addition to the project's quality evaluation (Akao et al. 1990).

Usually, QFD is used to express relationships between needs and characteristics (Mincolelli et al. 2020a, 2020b; Zairi and Youssef 1995). However, due to the finalities of the previously described analysis, in this specific project, it was decided to substitute characteristics with the designed sensory cues. This process aimed to select the most effective ones that would be then used for the subsequent trial.

In the following table, are listed all the needs obtained from the qualitative and quantitative analysis. For every need, a code was assigned, it was mentioned the typology of the user who expressed it, and, especially for the quantitative ones, it was declared the related parameter.

It is important to specify that the testing protocols collected many more parameters than the ones listed in this chapter. The multidisciplinary group analyzed them and chose the ones that could be put in relationship with the needs expressed by the project users (Table 6.1).

As previously described, the QFD matrix lines were filled with the obtained users' needs, while the columns reported all the cues used in the testing protocol.

Needs were then classified with a specific code and listed from the qualitative ones to the quantitative ones. Moreover, each need was evaluated with a score representing its absolute importance. Coherently with the traditional QFD used by industrial companies (Zairi and

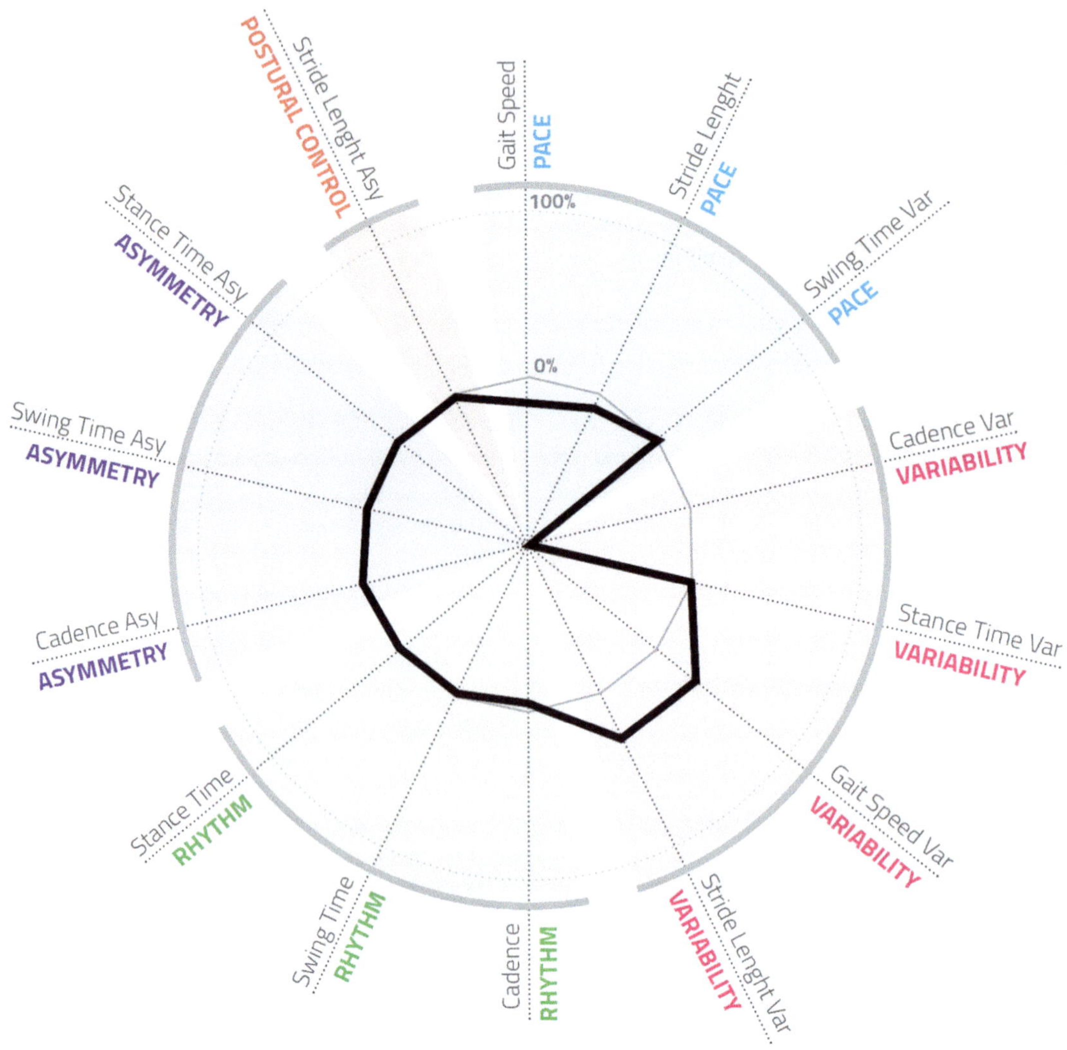

Fig. 6.10 Radar scheme showing collected parameters about the performance with visual cues submission

Youssef 1995; Francis 2016), the working group assigned a score from 1 to 5, representing the evaluation of every need's relevance within the research project's objectives.

Then, the QFD algorithm calculated percentages describing the needs' relative importance in comparison with the other ones in the matrix.

At this point of the process, the team was called to give a score expressing how much every cue could influence the user's gait, satisfying each specific need. The obtained scores were inserted into the boxes of intersection between lines and columns, following this classification:

0 (light gray): The cue does not respond to the need

1 (light pink): The cue weakly responds to the need

3 (pink): The cue satisfactorily responds to the need

9 (magenta): The cue strongly responds to the need

The additional use of colors improve the researchers' comprehension, even for those people not having an expertise in applying and

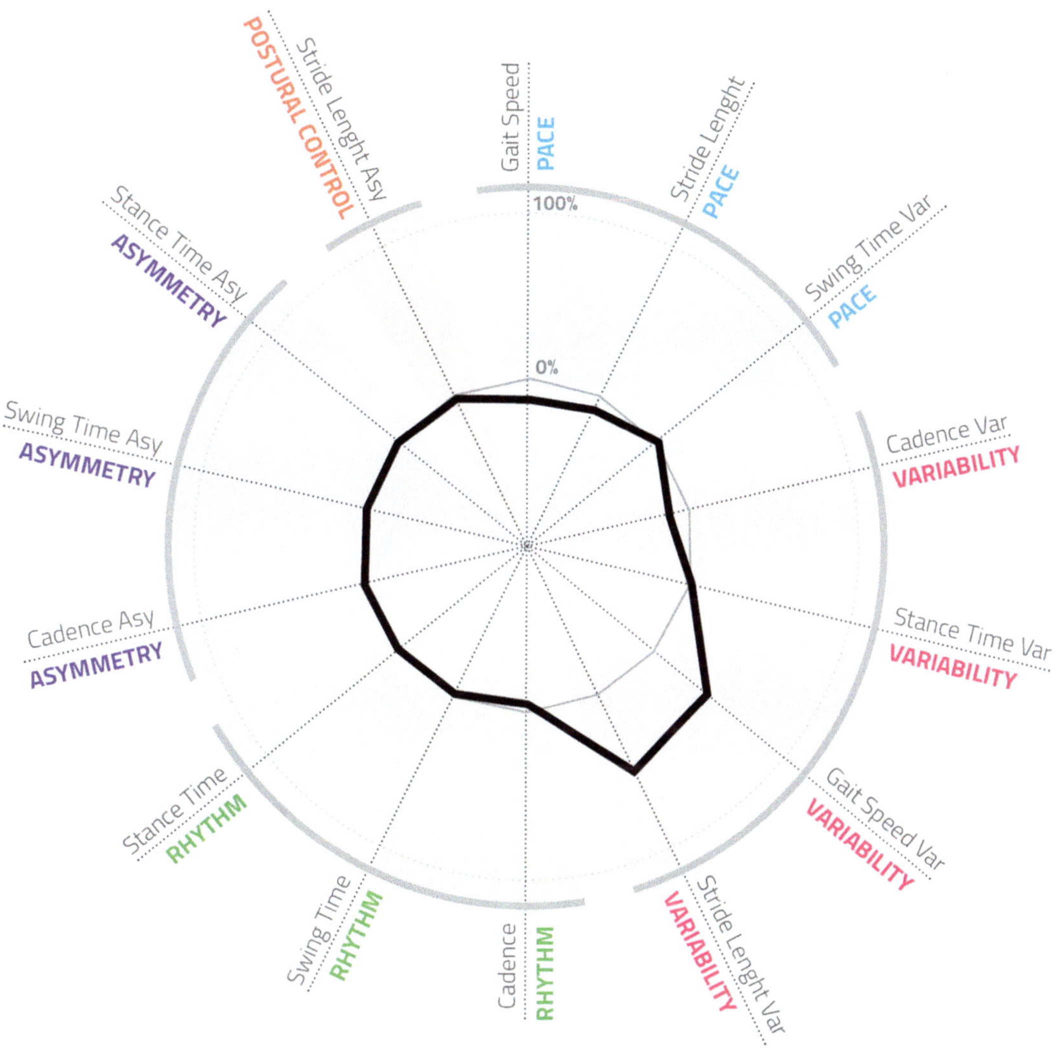

Fig. 6.11 Radar scheme showing collected parameters about the performance with auditory cues submission

interpreting the QFD matrix (Mincolelli et al. 2018) (Fig. 6.14).

The last two lines of the matrix showed values, elaborated by QFD algorithms, representing the needs' absolute and relative importance combined with scores about the signals' level of provided satisfaction. The line representing the needs' absolute importance reported values about actual cues' effectiveness, expressing how relevant was every analyzed qualitative and quantitative factor (Francis 2016). The last line expressing the percentage value of relative importance consents to an easy observation and interpretation of results of the different submitted sensory cues.

From the QFD degree of correlation between users' needs and sensory signals, the team obtained a hierarchization of the cues used during the testing protocol, matching all positive aspects and positive performances: B3, B2, B5, B1, B4, C2, C1, D3, A5, D1, D2, A1, A2, A3, A4, A6.

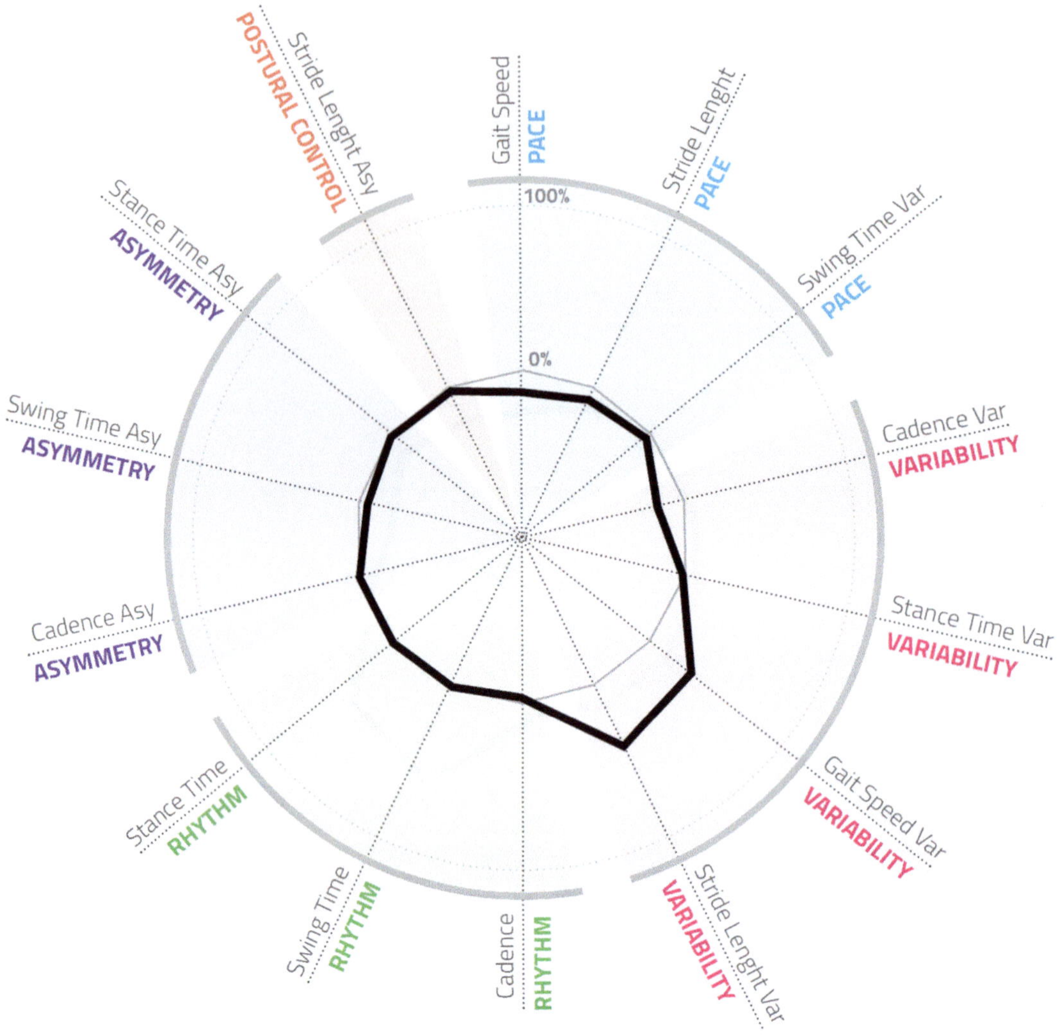

Fig. 6.12 Radar scheme showing collected parameters about the performance with vibratory cues submission

Results of the QFD Matrix

The first three tests (*Z1*, *Z2*, *Z3*) were performed without providing information to the user either on the type of signal that would receive or on the behavior that he/she would have to adapt to verify the perceptual impact of cues with the least possible conditioning.

Interestingly, the results suggested that the participants implicitly approached the rhythm imposed by the unimodal feedback. Furthermore, their cadence variability appears to be reduced compared to their reference walk, while the other spatio-temporal gait parameters seem to be invariant (Fig. 6.15).

Considering the classification finally expressed by the QFD matrix, it was possible to observe that cues were grouped in homogeneous sensory categories, even if singularly evaluated.

Auditory cues were the most effective ones, then the vibratory ones followed by the multisensory, and last, there were visual cues.

Considering the winning auditory channels, it is interesting to notice that the traditional metronome (B1) gained the result of 9%,

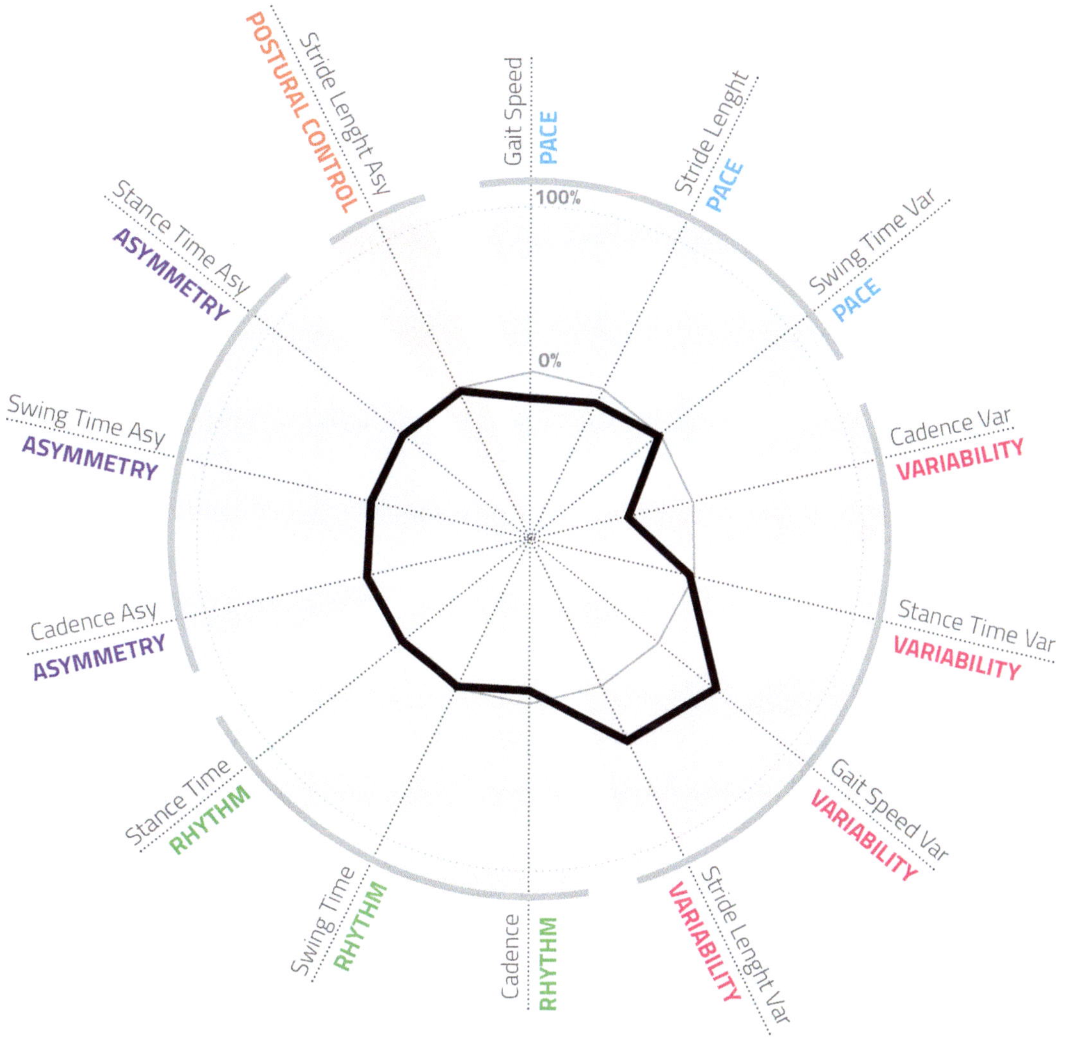

Fig. 6.13 Radar scheme showing collected parameters about the performance with multi-sensory cues submission

the lowest percentage among auditory signals. Besides, with 11% the winner was the melody played with musical instruments and electronic sounds (B3). The users perceived this last cue as less bothering in comparison with the metronome, and users were able to adapt to the target cadence with fewer steps. Signals reporting traditional musical instruments were considered by users as less annoying and calmer, thanks to their similarity to human natural sounds.

Vibratory cues were demonstrated to be not as effective as the auditory, gaining results similar to the ones of the metronome. Differently, signals transmitted only by the SG on the user's temple significantly limited the potential of cues acting with the haptic channel. Interestingly auditory and vibratory stimuli reduce the user's cadence variability, which is consistently elevated in people with PD (Peterson and Horak 2016).

Visual cues had the lowest performance: the reason seemed to be that this cue typology is better perceived if related to space perception, instead is not appropriate to provide temporal information, such as the cadence.

Table 6.1 Needs for the QFD matrix

Code	Need	User expressing the need	Kind of feedback	Related parameter
US01	I don't want it to be invasive and annoying	Test User	Qualitative	Interview
TO01	If it is invasive and annoying, I want all users to perceive it in the same way	Technical operator	Qualitative	Interview
US02	I don't want it to be difficult to follow the suggested rhythm	Test User	Qualitative	Interview
TO02	If it is difficult to align to the signal, I want all users to perceive it in the same way	Technical operator	Qualitative	Interview
TO03	I want the user's cadence to align with the target one	Technical operator	Quantitative	Difference between users' cadence and the target one
TO04	I want all users to have the same cadence when they receive the signal	Technical operator	Quantitative	Difference between users' cadence and the target one
TO05	I want the user to reach the target with a few steps	Technical operator	Quantitative	Number of steps to align to the rhythm
TO06	I want all users to reach the target cadence with the same amount of steps	Technical operator	Quantitative	Number of steps to align to the rhythm
TO07	I want the user to reduce the cadence variance in his gait	Technical operator	Quantitative	Cadence variability
TO08	I want the user's gait to be more balanced and symmetrical in right and left cadence	Technical operator	Quantitative	Asymmetry index on cadence
TO09	I want the user's gait to be more balanced and symmetrical in stride length	Technical operator	Quantitative	Asymmetry index on stride length

However, all the cues designed in this cycle seemed to bring the user to a more symmetrical gait in comparison with the baseline trial, endorsing the effective application of the cueing strategy.

Referring to scientific literature regarding multisensory feedback for gait analysis and training, it is known that different cueing modalities have differential effects on gait rehabilitation: while visual cueing primarily improves spatial gait parameters (e.g. stride length), auditory and haptic cueing mainly improve temporal gait parameters (e.g. gait speed and cadence) (Sigrist et al. 2013; Spaulding et al. 2013). The QFD outcomes are aligned with the previous considerations: all the auditory and vibratory feedback reach a higher percentage than the visual ones.

Moreover, the obtained results showed that the mono-sensory feedback is more performing than the multi-sensory signal, which sometimes was perceived by the users as annoying and overwhelming. The reason for the mono-sensory signals' success could be motivated by the application of a simple walking paradigm, where the user walked on a straight path without obstructions, training the adaptation to the suggested cadence. Differently, considering a complex motor task, multisensory cues could be applied

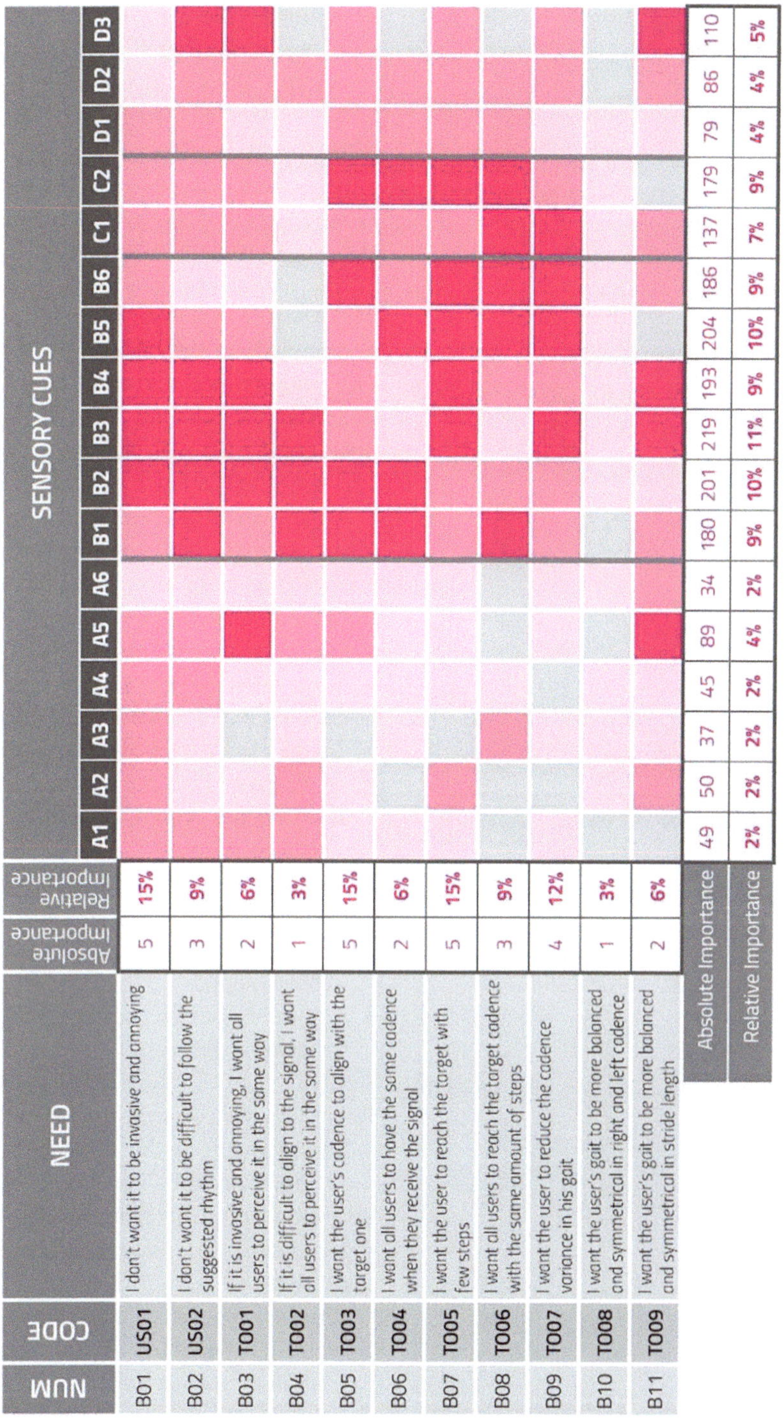

Fig. 6.14 Innovative use of the Quality Function Deployment matrix as a tool to determine the most effective sensory feedback submitted to the users

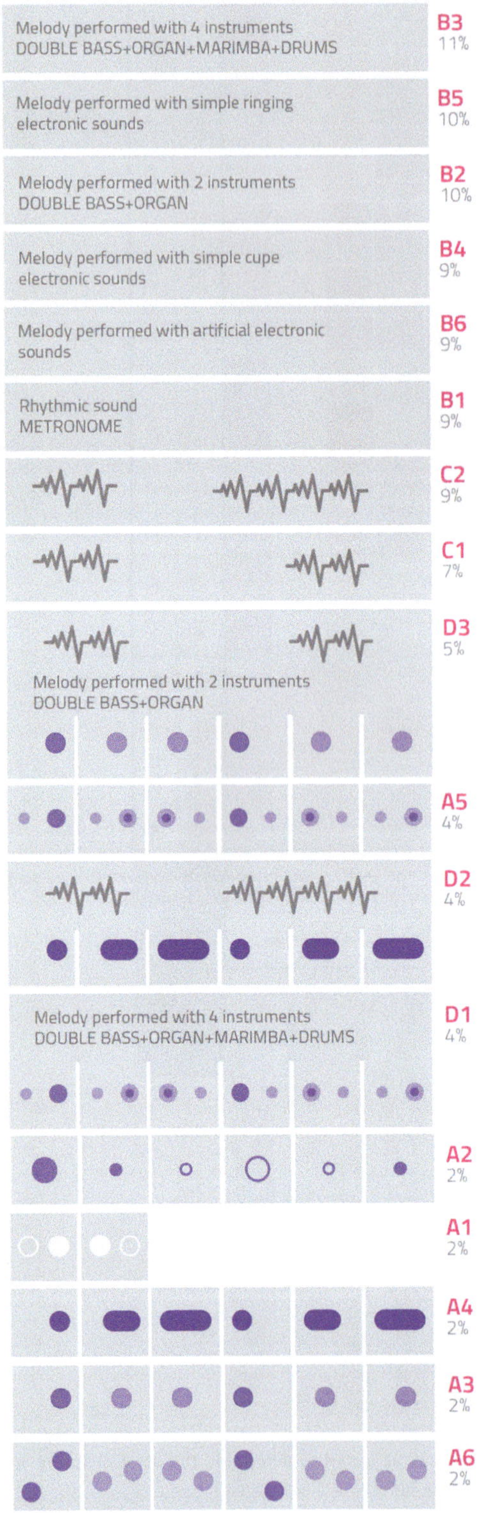

Fig. 6.15 Graphical representation of the cues, listed following QFD final results

to optimize the specific advantages of every typology of cues, such as the aptitude to visualize display alerts or spatial aspects, and of sound or haptic feedback to display temporal aspects (Sigrist et al. 2013).

6.3 Conclusions

This chapter describes the final part of the first design cycle of the PASSO project. Several visual, auditory, and vibratory cues were tested to understand which ones were more performing in conditioning the gait of tested users, adapting it to a suggested cadence.

Below are listed some summary statements about sensory cues deriving from the previous analysis that were used as guidelines for the next designing phase:

- Cues should always have a fixed point not moving in animations.
- Images in A cues should modify their color or dimension but not position.
- Cues should present images changing only in part their position.
- In A cues the movement of elements should be only horizontal.
- D cues should be composed of simple monosensory signals.
- D cues should be composed of simple monosensory signals.

Regarding visual cues, it was noticed that their submission forces the user to concentrate the view both on the signal and the path. This operation could be perceived as a bit confusing and can moderately compromise the user's performance.

Considering visual cues' ability to influence movements' spatiality rather than temporality (as auditory and somatosensory cues), it was decided to design visual cues usable to submit a task or a warning/alert regarding the path to the user. In this case, visual cues would deliver a punctual message instead of suggesting a rhythm to follow for a significant amount of steps.

Another strength of this new mHealth system was the common Android-based platform that allowed agile and real-time communication between the SG app and the system.

Identified critical points were the synchronization between the signal submission and the person's gait phase, the gap between the user's cadence and the one proposed by the system, and the location of the haptic cue limited to the right or left SG's temples.

Another limitation of the described approach concerned the extent to which each subject is visual-, auditory-, or somatosensory-dependent: the nervous system uses augmented sensory information differently, depending primarily on individual proclivities to rely on one sensory channel over another to control motor behavior.

To overcome some of these limitations, in the following testing phases, the target cadence was supposed to be subject-specific. In particular, during gait training, the target cadence should be based on the one detected during a user's reference gait. Alternatively, to comply with the therapeutic needs, the target cadence should be a modified version of the one recorded during the user's reference gait.

Finally, questionnaires and automated assessment methods should be used to evaluate patients' sensory preferences to empower their performance due to their abilities and attitudes.

The results of this first UCD design cycle were satisfactory and encouraging for the following cycles. In particular, the QFD tool's results confirmed the role of sensory cues on gait rehabilitation: auditory and haptic cues reach a higher efficacy than visual one; while visual cue improves spatial gait parameters (e.g., stride length), auditory and somatosensory stimuli improve temporal gait features (e.g., cadence).

The outcomes obtained in the first design cycle will be used in the design phases of cycle 2 (C2P1) and cycle 3 (C3P1), designing other system elements that will help achieve the purposes of the PASSO project.

Besides, the experimented UCD methodological process, especially the verifying phase (C1P4), was demonstrated to be effective in reducing the complexity of managing multidisciplinary design processes considering both human and technological aspects that are usually difficult to compare. This design strategy seems to be usable even in other typologies of inclusive research projects addressed to niche users with specific needs, providing a novel contribution to the field of simplification tools for the collection and combination of parameters allowing the evaluation of potential design solutions.

References

Y. Akao, G.H. Mazur, B. King, *Quality function deployment: integrating customer requirements into product design* (1990)

F. Francis, Engineering approach with quality function deployment for an ABET accredited program: a case study. Am. J. Mech. Eng. **4**(2), Art. no. 2 (2016). https://doi.org/10.12691/ajme-4-2-4

S. Imbesi, M. Corzani, Multisensory cues for gait rehabilitation with smart glasses: methodology, design, and results of a preliminary pilot. Sensors **23**(2), Art. no. 2 (2023). https://doi.org/10.3390/s23020874

S. Imbesi, G. Mincolelli, Design of a rehabilitation system monitoring gait of users with Parkinson's disease: data visualization as a methodological tool, in *Digital Human Modeling and Applied Optimization*, AHFE Open Acces (2022).https://doi.org/10.54941/ahfe1001907

G. Mincolelli, M. Marchi, S. Imbesi, Inclusive design for ageing people and the internet of things: understanding needs, in *Advances in Design for Inclusion*, G. Di Bucchianico, P.F. Kercher, Eds., in Advances in Intelligent Systems and Computing. Cham: Springer International Publishing, pp. 98–108 (2018). https://doi.org/10.1007/978-3-319-60597-5_9.

G. Mincolelli, S. Imbesi, M. Zallio, Collaborative quality function deployment. A methodology for enabling co-design research practice, in *Advances in Design for Inclusion*, G. Di Bucchianico, Ed., in Advances in Intelligent Systems and Computing. Cham: Springer International Publishing, pp. 91–99. https://doi.org/10.1007/978-3-030-20444-0_9

G. Mincolelli, G.A. Giacobone, M. Marchi, S. Imbesi, New collaborative version of the quality function deployment: practical application to the HABITAT project, in *Intelligent Human Systems Integration 2020*, T. Ahram, W. Karwowski, A. Vergnano, F. Leali, and R. Taiar, Eds., in Advances in Intelligent Systems and Computing. Cham: Springer International Publishing, pp. 823–828 (2020). https://doi.org/10.1007/978-3-030-39512-4_125

D.S. Peterson, F.B. Horak, Neural control of walking in people with parkinsonism. Physiol. Bethesda

Md 31(2), 95–107 (2016). https://doi.org/10.1152/physiol.00034.2015
R. Sigrist, G. Rauter, R. Riener, P. Wolf, Augmented visual, auditory, haptic, and multimodal feedback in motor learning: a review. Psychon. Bull. Rev. 20(1), 21–53 (2013). https://doi.org/10.3758/s13423-012-0333-8
S.J. Spaulding, B. Barber, M. Colby, B. Cormack, T. Mick, M.E. Jenkins, Cueing and gait improvement among people with Parkinson's disease: a meta-analysis. Arch. Phys. Med. Rehabil. 94(3), 562–570 (2013). https://doi.org/10.1016/j.apmr.2012.10.026
M. Zairi, M.A. Youssef, Quality function deployment: a main pillar for successful total quality management and product development. Int. J. Qual. Reliab. Manag. 12(6), 9–23 (1995). https://doi.org/10.1108/02656719510089894

Cycle 2: Smart Devices for Cues' Submission

7

Abstract

The PASSO project is composed of three design cycles, this chapter describes in detail the phases of the second cycle, dedicated to the design of an innovative smart device for the submission of haptic cues to people affected by Parkinson's disease. During the planning phase, the multidisciplinary team defined users and stakeholders, and the project context; in the analyzing phase users' needs were collected and an analysis of devices submitting haptic cues was conducted; in the creating phase, it was applied the Quality Function Deployment tool, and several design solutions were developed and prototyped; finally, during the verifying phase, the prototyped were tested to collect quantitative and qualitative data for the validation of this part of the research project.

7.1 Structure of Cycle 2

The second design cycle of the PASSO project aimed to develop a wearable smart device transmitting sensory cues to the user during the user's training (Fig. 7.1). Specifically, in this cycle, a novel smart device was tested for the transmission of haptic cues exerting vibrations over specific parts of the body able to correct the posture of the user making him less unbalanced in the frontal and mediolateral plans. The research questions faced in this part of the PASSO project were: How many actuators should have the device? Where should they be positioned? Is it possible to train people to improve posture with vibrations?

During the previous cycle, analyzing how sensory cues can influence gait parameters to practice a specific rehabilitation program, users received signals submitted by SG lenses for visual cues, earphones for auditory, and SG temples for vibratory ones.

Considering that visual cues were considered suitable only to give spatial feedback, and that no negative aspects were detected using earphones for auditory cues and vibrations transmitted by SG temples, these were defined the signals with broader possibilities of improvement (Imbesi et al. 2021a).

The second cycle aimed to analyze, design, and test a smart device primarily focused on transmitting vibrations to the person's body to improve gait and posture (including Pisa syndrome and forward lean of the trunk) (Imbesi et al. 2022).

To overcome some of the limitations raised during the first cycle, in the second one the target cadence was supposed to be subject-specific. In particular, the target cadence should be based on the one detected during a user's reference gait during gait training. Alternatively, to comply with the therapeutic needs, the target cadence should be a modified version of the one recorded during the user's reference gait.

S. Imbesi, *Inclusive Design of a Smart Device for People with Parkinson's Disease*, Design For Inclusion 4, https://doi.org/10.1007/978-3-031-58249-3_7

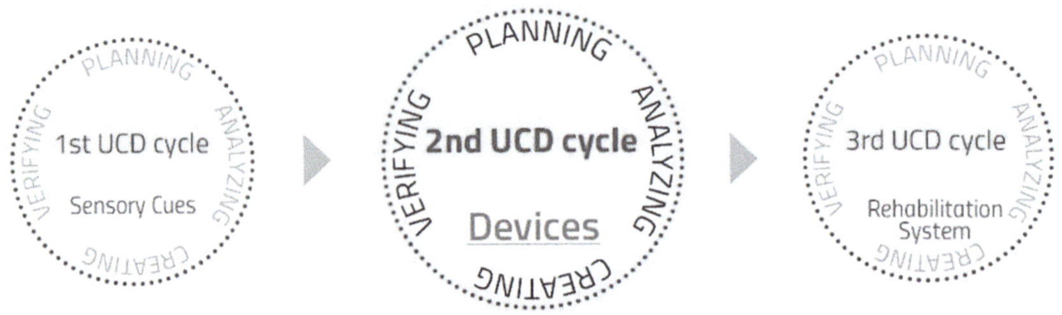

Fig. 7.1 Schematization of the user-centered iterative design cycles

Finally, questionnaires or automated assessment methods should evaluate patients' sensory preferences to empower their performance due to their abilities and attitudes.

7.2 Planning Phase (C2P1)

This design cycle used the same mix of multidisciplinary competencies as the previous cycle. Indeed, the included professionalisms were:

- Designers (user research, usability, UCD methodology, interaction design, product design, visual design, etc.);
- Technical operators (biomedical engineering, computer science and technology, informatics, etc.);
- Medical operators (neurology, physiatry, physiotherapy, geriatrics, etc.).

Users identified and engaged in this project cycle were:

- PD USER (US): A user is the PD person involved in this project. Typically he/she is facing the early stages of the disease, trying to contrast this degeneration thanks to different typologies of cognitive and motor rehabilitation and training, under the observation and cure of a specialized doctor.
- MEDICAL OPERATOR (MO): Medical operators involved in this design cycle specialized in physiatrists addressed to patients affected by PD. They usually carry out trials, experimenting with new devices for their training sessions. Usually, they practice rehabilitation on persons' gait and posture, to postpone or decelerate motor symptoms.
- TECHNICAL OPERATOR (TO): The technical operators engaged in this project cycle were a designer, a biomedical engineer, an ICT engineer, and an informatician. They belonged to the multidisciplinary team developing the PASSO project.

According to the scientific literature about smart devices for the submission of sensory cues specifically submitting haptic signals to the user's trunk, the use of vibrotactile stimuli shown to bring an improvement in people's walking performances, tested in several environments by different users (Gonçalves et al. 2021). Besides, haptic cues do not engage fine physical capabilities that could be invalidated by aging, like vision and hearing (Reich and Savitt 2019). For these reasons, it would be desirable to experiment with vibratory cues in applications like improving balance or avoiding falls, in addition to Freezing Of the Gait (FOG) contrast (Davie 2008; Nieuwboer 2008). For the submission of this typology of signal, IMU was integrated into the smart wearable device. Commonly, inertial sensors are positioned in the ankle, lower trunk, knees, shins, hip, and plantar (Gonçalves et al. 2021). In analyzing biofeedback systems based on vibrotactile feedback working specifically on balance, the most common placement is the trunk area, precisely at the waist level (Lee et al. 2018).

To transmit the vibrating signal, the multidisciplinary team chose to use as sensors and actuators some Smart Watches (SW) fastened to a wearable cloth keeping them positioned in the correct part of the person's body.

To test the system primarily in an ambulatory context several prototypes were developed with the supervision and support of a medical operator; in further developments, the system should be usable even by users in their everyday environments performing daily activities, both indoor and outdoor.

7.3 Analyzing Phase (C2P2)

The analyzing phase considered users' needs as human factors determining the research project's requirements, and the characteristics of technologies as technical constraints influencing the choice of solutions for the prototypes development.

Needs Collection

Due to collecting users' needs, some individual informal interviews were submitted (Mincolelli et al. 2018). Specifically, individual talks were organized with users previously described: PD users (US), medical operators (MO), and technical operators (TO).

Collected needs were grouped according to the domain they refer to Imbesi and Scataglini (2021). The list of domains was elaborated starting from a list describing the widespread needs of older users about smart garments.

In the following table are listed needs collected during the interviews, each need was defined as a code and specified which user it was addressed to Imbesi and Mincolelli (2020) (Table 7.1).

Analysis of Devices for the Submission of Haptic Cues

Postural control regards maintaining, achieving, and restoring balance during movements (Pollock et al. 2000). Some aspects of postural control are impaired in people with PD and affect their gait (Peterson and Horak 2016). Considering that maintaining balance during walking or standing tasks requires precise control of the head-arms-trunk (HAT) segments (Biomechanics and Motor Control of Human Movement, 2021), people with PD showed while standing increased area, velocity, and jerkiness of postural sway and reduced stability limits, defined as the maximum center of mass displacement possible without changing one's base of support. The characteristic flexed, inflexible postural alignment of people with PD results in a forward position of the body center of mass, possibly to protect against backward falling (Schieppati and Nardone 1991). Lateral balance control is particularly affected as lateral trunk sway is significantly high during quiet stance (Adkin et al. 2005; Mancini et al. 2012) and while walking with and without obstacles (Galna et al. 2013; Stegemöller et al. 2012). While a small amount of lateral movement is necessary for stability and optimized energetics (Kuo and Donelan 2010), too much lateral movement is likely harmful and is related to increased falls (Rogers and Mille 2003).

Thus, providing information about trunk sway to patients could help enhance their postural control; one way to realize this is via artificial biofeedback systems that supplement natural sensory inputs, providing additional sensory information about trunk inclination to the brain (Woollacott et al. 1993).

Sensors' location needs to be considered a crucial part of the design process in light of its impact on the wearability of the system. According to Gonçalves et al., a scientific literature review about wearable devices submitting haptic feedback shows that the most commonly chosen location for the sensor is the ankle zone, or waist, shins, and foot insole, whether actuators are usually separately located in a different body area like head, trunk, waist, hip, wrist, ankle and foot insole (Gonçalves et al. 2021).

Regarding actuators transmitting the vibratory cue, the multidisciplinary team tested which part of the trunk was more suitable for their

Table 7.1 Users' needs listed by typology

Category of requirement	Code	Need	User expressing the need
Aesthetics anxiety	US01	I don't want other people to perceive it	PD user
	US02	I don't want it to seem like a medical device	PD user
	US03	I want to put and remove it without help	PD user
Comfort	US04	I want it to be in a material I feel comfortable with	PD user
	US05	I don't want it to reduce my mobility	PD user
	US06	I want it to be my size	PD user
	TO01	I want to be able to change the size for every user I test	Technical operator
	MO01	I want it to be adaptable to different users' sizes	Medical operator
Functionality issues	US09	I want it to last as long as I need it	PD user
	US10	I want to be able to activate it by myself	PD user
	US11	I don't want the equipment to suddenly stop functioning	PD user
	TO02	I don't want smartwatches to risk to follow	Technical operator
	TO03	I don't want it to have atypical or unexpected functionalities	Technical operator
	TO04	I don't want smartwatches to move accidentally after the positioning	Technical operator
	TO05	I want the user to perceive the signal	Technical operator
	MO02	I want to set the target correction angle for every patient	Medical operator
	MO03	I want it to impact on the most disabling postural impairment	Medical operator
Technology anxiety	US12	I don't want to be apprehensive about using it	PD user
	US13	I don't want to worry about breaking it	PD user
	US14	I don't want it to interfere with other aids or devices (e.g. pacemaker, hearing aids, and others)	PD user
	TO06	I want it to be compatible and integrable with Android systems	Technical operator
Perceived ubiquity	US15	I want it to provide me with anytime and anywhere communication and connectivity	PD user
	TO07	I want it to monitor parameters every time the user is wearing it	Technical operator
	MO04	I want to use it for healthcare and well-being purposes	Medical operator
Resistance	US16	I don't want it to change the way I interact with other people	PD user
	US17	I don't want it to change the way I currently live	PD user
	MO05	I don't want to disappoint the user in training	Medical operator
Perceived usefulness	US18	I want it to improve my life quality	PD user
	US19	I want it to make my life more convenient	PD user
	US20	I want it to make me more effective in my life	PD user
Perceived ease of use	US21	I want it to be easy to use ara>	PD user
	US22	I don't want it to require a lot of mental effort	PD user
	MO06	I don't want to make her/him feel inadequate during the training	Medical operator
Attitude	US23	I want to think that it is beneficial to me	PD user
	US24	I want to have a positive perception of using it	PD user
	US25	I want it to make me feel safe	PD user
	MO07	I don't want to frighten her/him by proponing the system testing protocol	Medical operator
Behavioral intention	US26	I want to use it in the future	PD user
	US27	I want to use it in my daily life	PD user
	US28	I want my parents to appreciate my improvements	PD user

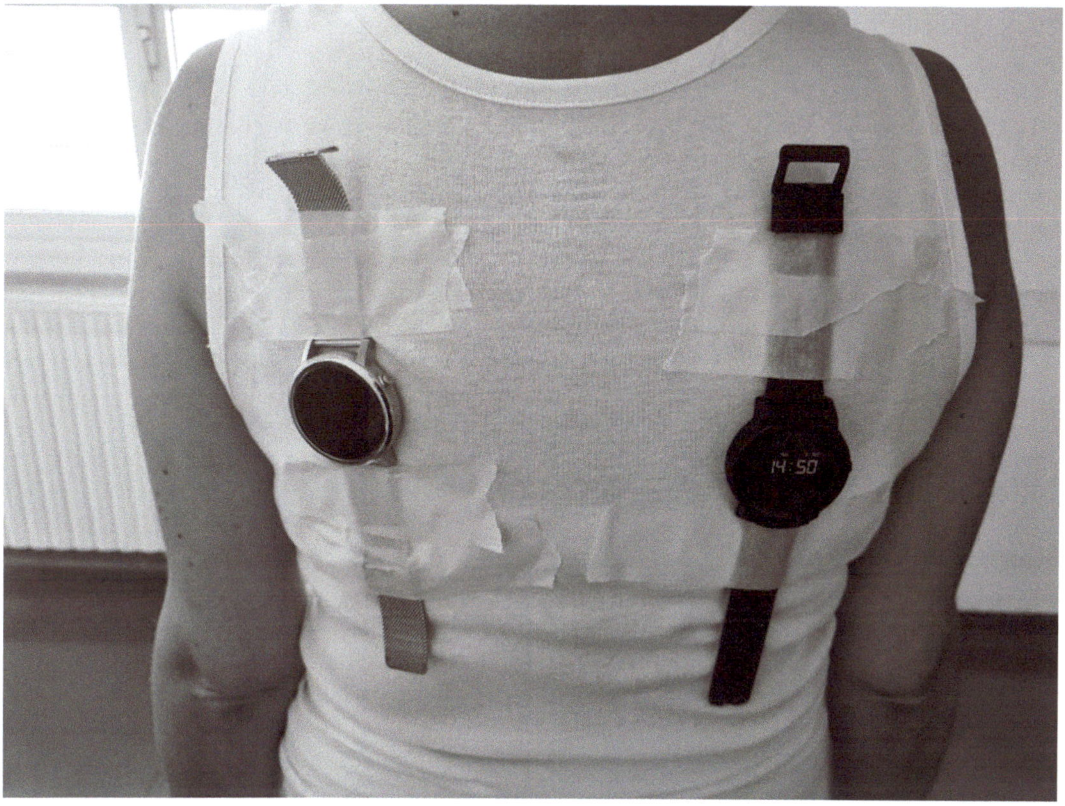

Fig. 7.2 Picture representing some of the evaluated solutions for actuators' positioning

location transmitting the signal near the bone structures, which could make it perceptible in a clear but not annoying way. Choosing a comfortable location, not stressing the user, was crucial in this project because of its impact on the device's usability.

Different options were evaluated to understand which stimulus location could be perceived as stronger and positively affect body posture, limiting the person's inclination on the frontal and mediolateral planes (Fig. 7.2).

7.4 Creating Phase (C2P3)

Thanks to considerations elaborated in the first phases of this design cycle, it was possible to select some needs expressed by users (PD person, technical operator, medical operator) and evaluate their degree of relationship with some of the characteristics attributed to the smart device, and the related system, developed in this design cycle (Imbesi et al. 2021b).

Quality Function Deployment

The Quality Function Deployment (QFD) tool was used in a modified version, aiming to improve the accessibility to all multidisciplinary team members (Mincolelli et al. 2020a). It maintained its primary objective of creating a hierarchy between the project's features and the users' needs (Akao and Mazur 2003).

This QFD matrix highlighted which technical characteristics had the most appreciable impact on the project's success (Zairi and Youssef 1995). Some measurable characteristics of the device and the system were selected to fill the QFD, with the help of technical operators involved in the project.

The whole team was then asked to assess a score to every need to choose the ones to be inserted in the matrix. After this step, the team attributed a mark to the degree of relationship between every need and every characteristic. The final scores were inserted in boxes of intersection between the matrix's lines and columns, according to the following scale:

0 (light gray): The cue does not respond to the need
1 (light pink): The cue weakly responds to the need
3 (pink): The cue satisfactorily responds to the need
9 (magenta): The cue strongly responds to the need

The QFD algorithm elaborated values of relative and absolute importance for considered characteristics, based on the marks previously collected (Fig. 7.3).

The colors used in the matrix boxes helped the reading and interpretation of obtained results, even for team members who were not experts in using the QFD matrix (Mincolelli et al. 2018).

QFD results were a significant reference for developing design and technical solutions (Mincolelli et al. 2020b). Results expressed a hierarchization of selected characteristics addressed to the device and the system (Table 7.2).

Interpreting QFD results, it was possible to notice that technical characteristics impacting more on the project's usability, in relationship with selected users (PD person, medical operator, technical operator), are the ones related to a possible personalization of the device's physical features and the system's settings. Even the number of actions requested to set the training and the correspondent user's autonomy in completing tasks proved its relevance.

The characteristics resulting as less impacting on the project's success were the device's weight, its energetic autonomy, and the cost of the whole system.

Developing Design and Technological Solutions

In light of the previous considerations, the multidisciplinary team decided not to primarily focus on the gait satisfactorily tested in the first design cycle but on postural control.

According to suggestions given by medical operators, the chosen points on the shoulders, back, and chest were supposed to straighten the user's trunk when pending forward and to lead to a correct posture when unbalanced on the lateral side (Fig. 7.4).

At the beginning of this part of the project, the intention was to design a sort of shirt incorporating the faces of smartwatches used as actuators transmitting the vibratory cue. While elaborating on previous considerations, it was clear that the solution needed to be improved: detected problems were the correct positioning of smartwatch faces on different body parts and the low pressure exerted by the fabric on the devices that did not guarantee the right contact with the body, weakening the perception of the signal.

To overcome these issues the author developed a tailored harness modifying a postural band for the shoulders and back. This solution guaranteed a more precise positioning of smartwatches, a higher pressure on the smartwatch's body, allowing their contact with the body, and, finally, concrete help to postural training in the light of its autonomous function of a corrective health device (Imbesi et al. 2022).

It was then considered to shift to a different kind of cloth embodying actuators: a tailored harness was developed, inspired by a postural band for shoulders and back.

Initially, three solutions for sensory cues were developed:

single short vibration,
single persistent vibration,
intermittent vibration.

After a first application with the medical operator, the single short intermittent vibration was chosen to correct pendency. The cue with the single persistent vibration was perceived as anesthetizing, so its use was stopped.

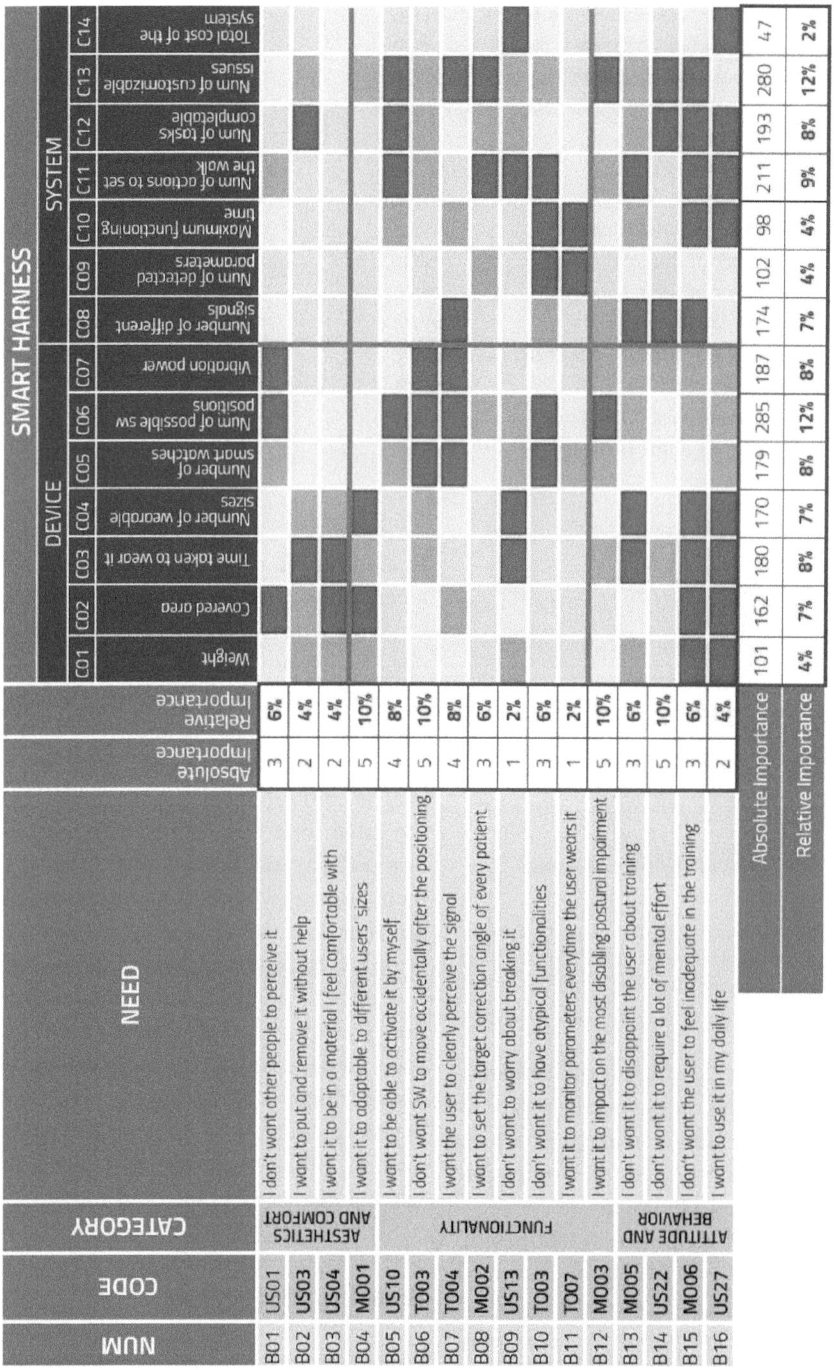

Fig. 7.3 Quality Function deployment matrix for the smart harness

Table 7.2 Final list of characteristics of importance

Code	Characteristic	Element	Relative importance	Absolute importance (%)
C06	Number of possible SW positions	Device	285	12
C13	Number of customizable settings	System	280	12
C11	Number of actions to set the walk	System	211	9
C12	Number of tasks completable autonomously	System	193	8
C07	Vibration power	Device	187	8
C03	Time taken to wear it	Device	180	8
C05	Number of smartwatches	Device	179	8
C08	Number of different signals	System	174	7
C04	Number of wearable sizes	Device	170	7
C02	Covered area	Device	162	7
C09	Number of detected parameters	Device	102	4
C01	Weight	Device	101	4
C10	Maximum functioning time	System	98	4
C14	Total cost of the system	System	47	2

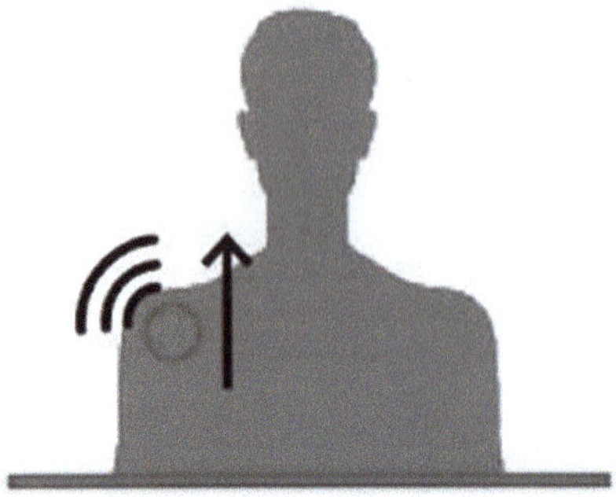

Fig. 7.4 When the cue was submitted to correct mediolateral inclination, it was observed that the vibration had the effect of lifting the affected shoulder

Analyzing possible positions of actuators transmitting the vibrating cues several positions were tested by the multidisciplinary group to understand which locations were most perceptible and less bothersome to the user.

For the correction of mediolateral inclination, as represented in Fig. 7.5, SW was positioned behind the shoulder's blade or over the shoulder. These locations consented to the proximity of the signal to the bones, allowing a better cue transmission.

Differently, to correct the frontal inclination, tested configurations used only one actuator located on the central part of the sternum, or in a central position on the back, as represented in schemes D and E in Fig. 7.6. The second developed solution considered the contemporary submission of three sensory cues behind the shoulder blade/over shoulders and on the chest/back, as represented in schemes F and G.

The solution involving three SWs vibrating at the same time was dismissed because perceived as too strong and bothersome. Finally, for frontal inclination, it was chosen to use a single actuator positioned in the central upper part of the chest or on the back between shoulder blades.

Considering the efficacy shown by both solutions, the choice of the harness model was left to users, depending on their personal preferences.

Developed solutions were used as inputs for the realization of several prototypes aiming at locating actuators in the best positions without making the user feel uncomfortable.

Building Prototypes

Developed design and technological solutions were used to develop two detailed prototypes inspired postural bands improving trunk posture thanks to a harness shape pushing shoulders back.

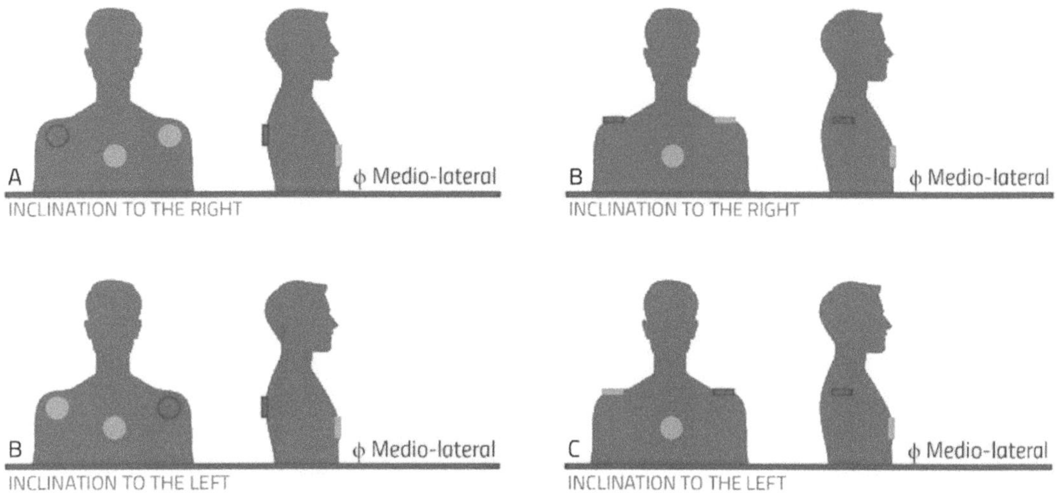

Fig. 7.5 Actuator positioning for the correction of mediolateral inclination

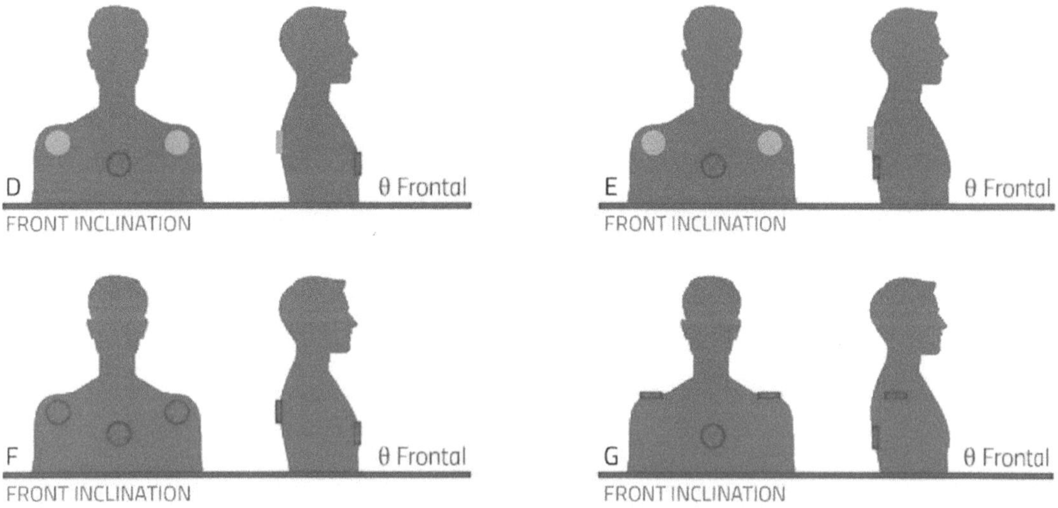

Fig. 7.6 Actuator positioning for the correction of frontal inclination

The first smart harness allowed up to three SW positions: the lateral ones on the shoulder blade or over the shoulder and the central one on the sternum. This solution was conceived for users who tend to unbalance only in the frontal plane, helping them reach a better posture by submitting a sensory signal. This configuration provided one vibration on the chest or three contemporary vibrations on the chest and shoulders (Fig. 7.7).

The second smart harness model differed from the first because it did not allow the frontal position of the central SW, which was instead located near the first thoracic vertebrae. This typology allowed a better posture for the person, increasing the effect offered by the postural band. This model was primarily created for people who tend to unbalance on the lateral plan, allowing different options for positioning the SW closer to the shoulder area (Fig. 7.8).

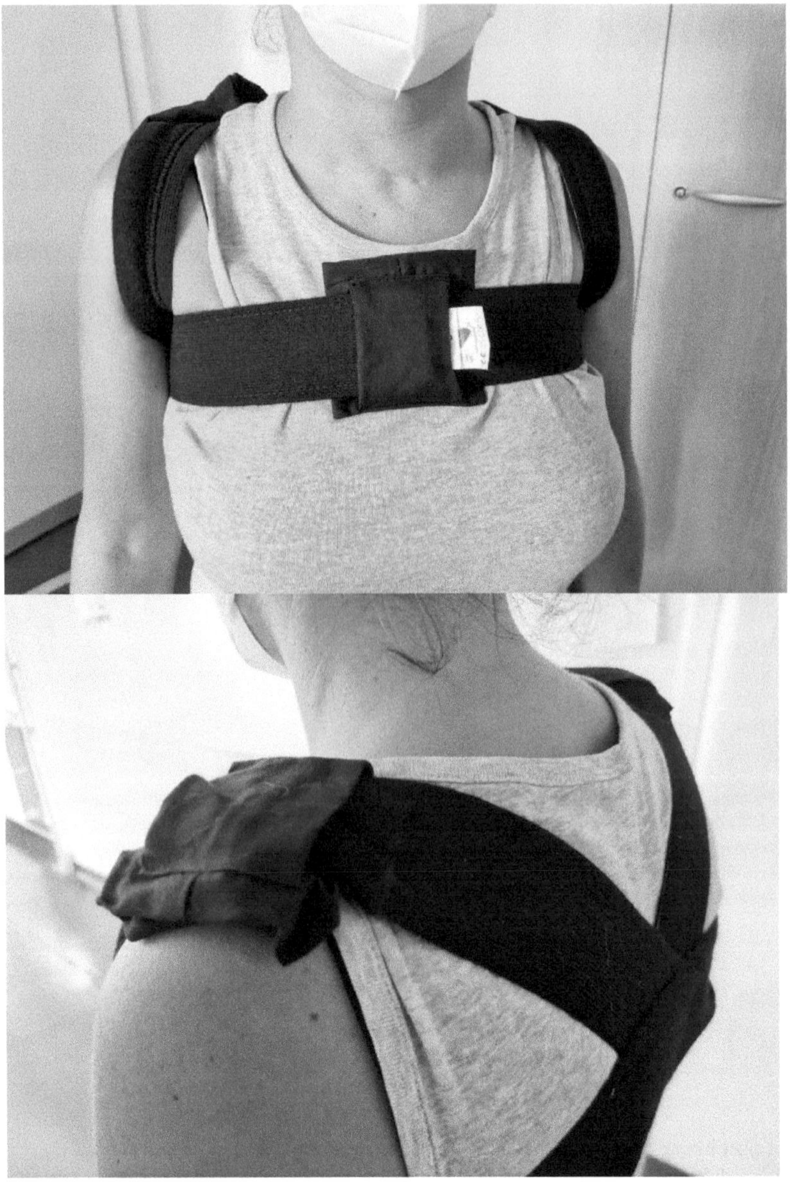

Fig. 7.7 First developed smart harness

Regarding the developed mHealth system, the remote control was exerted by a smartphone, setting the possible modalities of use and starting/stopping the SW's functions (Fig. 7.9).

When settings were selected, the operator could start the patient's training. The system guided the user with voice instructions: initially, it reminded the subject to maintain their target posture; subsequently, once this first phase of calibration was completed, the system warned the user that he could start walking. Thus, based on the set threshold, the SW submitted the corrective haptic feedback to help the subject return to the reference position (Imbesi et al. 2022).

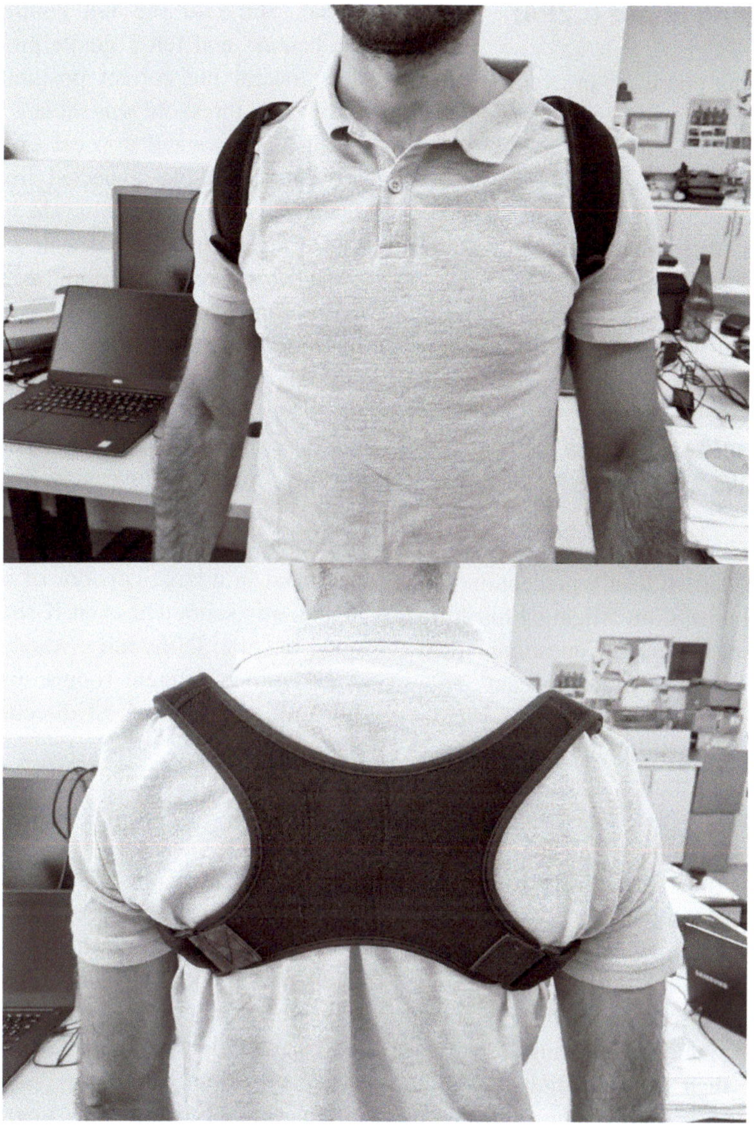

Fig. 7.8 Second developed smart harness

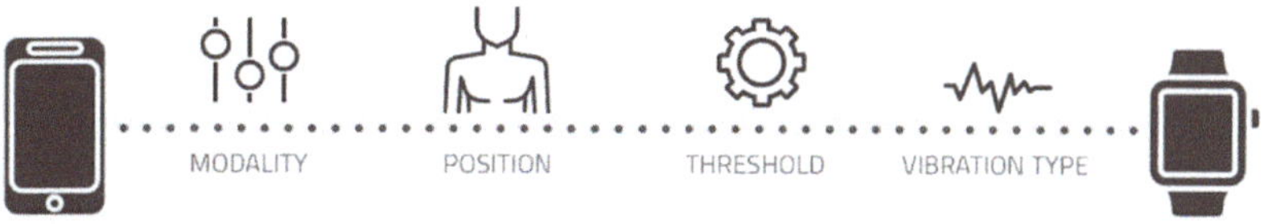

Fig. 7.9 Scheme representing the developed mHealth system

7.5 Verifying Phase (C2P4)

This last verifying phase, as in cycle 1, wanted to collect qualitative and quantitative information to evaluate the effectiveness and usability of the designed system.

This phase involved PD users in the experimentation, and their participation was fundamental to testing the developed device functioning only in the presence of real posture impairments.

Collecting Qualitative Data with Interviews

Qualitative data were collected with an individual interview about the user's perception of the tested postural harness, investigating his attitude toward the device. The open questionnaire was composed of the following questions:

- How do you feel wearing the smart harness?
- Is there something that makes you uncomfortable?
- Do you feel it leads you to a better posture?
- How do you think your walk has changed after the stimuli received?

Some users participated in the project giving their availability to sessions of discussion with operators, analyzing and wearing prototypes, and explaining their considerations about the whole project aspects. The main significant ones are described below.

User with PD (1)
She is 72, and she has a lateral inclination on the right side. She is very positive and open to new typologies of training and rehabilitation. She is a little abundant, she didn't practice sports in her life but likes to walk and train herself.

She felt more comfortable testing the second smart harness (back one) due to her large breasts. She chose the configuration with the horizontal smartwatch on the right shoulder because it allowed her a better perception of the vibrating signal. She said she felt comfortable wearing the harness and felt a gentle push of the shoulders toward the correct postural position. The right angle threshold was set at 8° and gave good results. She wanted a vocal explanation of the movement that we expected from her because she felt insecure about what she had to do.

During her performance, it was very easy to see when she received submitted signals because every time she had a visible reaction in the interested shoulder that quickly lifted up. She strongly wanted to do a good job, asking about the system functioning and deeply understanding how she was supposed to behave during the submission of vibratory cues.

She lamented that when she turned on herself to change direction in the right path (180°) and practiced in a large corridor of the hospital, the signal was submitted even if she felt she had a good posture. Differently, when she practiced a walk among different rooms simulating a real-life task, soft changes of direction didn't cause alarms.

She was satisfied with her performance with the system.

User with PD (2)
He is aged 62 and has very little frontal inclination of the trunk. He is a little shy but curious and open-minded. He has an extremely sporty physique as he practiced many years of athletics. He currently likes long walks on the hills in not-too-steep terrain.

Andrea tested the first smart harness (chest one), and he said he felt comfortable. The medical operator, after a few trials, tested his angle threshold at 5°.

Despite the very low value of the threshold, it was very satisfying to see it work. He was very interested in the functioning of the system, he made a lot of questions and comparisons with the other rehabilitation systems that he was using with satisfaction.

He didn't have visible reactions but felt the vibration and corrected his posture. He lamented, as Vanna, that when he turned sometimes the smartwatch vibrated.

After this first trial, he proposed to test even the lateral configuration because in this period he felt the right shoulder lower than the other. He chose the positioning behind the shoulder blade. A 3-degree angle was set as a threshold and felt the vibration a few times.

In both configurations, Andrea was very satisfied with his performance and curious about future developments.

Medical Operator
She is 42 years old, and she is a physiatrist working on patients in the first stages of PD. She is involved in scientific research and enjoys taking part in experimental projects that can potentially make her work more effective. She is a positive, attentive, and caring person with her patients, by whom she is particularly appreciated.

She has been the first person to experiment with prototypes and give advice for their implementation. She wanted to be sure about the devices' usability before using them with her patients.

She simulated the impairments she wanted to train and tested all possible configurations of the system. She gave precious advice for the development of final solutions and found the patients she thought best suited for the more in-depth meetings and interviews.

Technical Operator
He is 32 and is a biomedical engineer working on Android system development. He programmed the features of the system designing it with the technical operator working on design aspects. Mattia was very involved in the project and carried out the testing phase with other users and operators, modifying the system in real-time in order to make obtained suggestions immediately testable.

Collecting Quantitative Data with the Testing Protocol

Otherwise, quantitative data were collected during a testing protocol involving users and operators in the developed prototypes' testing.

Operators collected every user's data such as age, height, and sex. Users' walks were filmed to have a gold standard for doubts (frame both the walking subject and the operator sending the stimulus).

The testing protocol was applied in an ambulatory context. The equipment consisted of a SW with the related smartphone (used by the technical operator) and the smart harness where the SW was inserted.

The medical operator involved in the testing protocol had to evaluate the person to set target trunk inclination angles adopted as standards for the person's correct walking posture. The technical operator set into the system the chosen thresholds.

The user was first asked to wear the model of the smart harness that the operators chose for him. He was then demanded to choose a favorite positioning on his shoulders in an area where he could perceive the signal clearly but not annoyingly.

The testing protocol was organized into several phases:

- 1-min standing test without cues
- 1-min standing test with cues
- 2 min walk without cues in a linear path
- 2 min walk with cues in a linear path
- 3 min walk with cues in real-life/ecological path.

At the beginning of the testing protocol, the person, helped by the medical operator, adopted the target position for a correct posture. The system was then switched on, detecting in five seconds the target trunk inclination in frontal and mediolateral plans.

Afterward, the user had to face the first 2 min of walking along an ambulatory corridor without submitting any vibratory cue.

Finally, during the second 2-min walk, the patient received a vibration every time his real-time Pitch and Roll angles overcame set ones.

The user performed the last walk of 3 min in a real-life context, including some obstacles and demanding tasks, such as taking turns, opening a door, taking an elevator, climbing stairs, and others.

Qualitative and Quantitative Evaluations About Design and Technology

After testing different configurations, it was observed that the best cues for clarity and ease of interpretation were the ones involving only a single SW at a time.

The reason for this choice is fundamentally linked to the clinician's priorities: for a PD patient it is important to define one and only one clinical target to improve his most impaired function. The contemporary attempt to correct more than one gait or posture aspect at the same time could make the user cognitively overwhelmed; on the contrary, the request of a single task allows the patient to focus only on that goal, making his performance more effective.

For example, for subjects with Pisa Syndrome, one SW on the compromised lateral side acting as a reminder every time needed is enough. In this way, the mHealth system developed is highly customizable and can better follow the clinical needs.

While testing prototypes with users, customization was confirmed as a fundamental issue to be considered in the project. The features of the two developed harness models were diversely perceived by different users, depending on their body shape. For example, it was clear that the smart harnesses needed to be adaptable to different users' sizes, and that some women did not feel comfortable wearing the solution with the band on the chest. Another observed aspect was the necessity of a model allowing different locations of smartwatches over and behind the shoulders, considering the different sensitivity of the user's skin and the individual fat mass.

Even the system was designed considering the possibility of different configurations in the smartwatch's location on the user's trunk.

7.6 Conclusions

As in the first design cycle, the multidisciplinary team observed that multiple stimulations can confuse the user and make him feel uncomfortable and overwhelmed. That is the reason why, after several proofs, it was finally decided to use only one SW at a time, correcting the different typologies of inclination one by one: when patients present an inclination both in the frontal and mediolateral plans, it is better to act only on the inclination evaluated as higher. Training the person in the correction of this singular aspect will lead to a consequent decrease even in the inclination in the other plane.

Personalization is fundamental in smart devices addressed to PD users. Used smart harnesses were adjustable in size, increasing the fit and wearability of the wearable device, but were also perceived differently by users, depending on their body. Even the positioning of the SW in the smart harness was not felt in the same way by people (in the case of frontal inclination most of the users preferred to have the SW positioned on the chest, but some others felt uncomfortable with this configuration and preferred the one with the SW on the back between shoulder blades).

Haptic cues, as described in scientific literature, shown to be performative in correcting the posture of people with PD. The innovative positioning of the vibrating stimulus on the upper part of the trunk was able to make users instinctively correct their posture without needing an explanation of what to do at the signal submission. This aspect seems very significant because it reduces the cognitive impact of the cue on the person, lowering the mental effort requested for the posture-demanded correction.

The UCD methodology led to satisfactory results: the users' participation in the design process allowed a huge contribution to the design of the device, which was finally perceived as comfortable, useful, and easy to use. The needs collection and the application of the QFD tool allowed the definition of characteristics most impacting on this design cycle, considered in the prototypes' development.

The obtained results are an original contribution to Inclusive Design Research addressed to PD users for the implementation of posture training protocols including the submission of sensory cues.

References

A.L. Adkin, B.R. Bloem, J.H.J. Allum, Trunk sway measurements during stance and gait tasks in Parkinson's disease. Gait Posture **22**(3), 240–249 (2005). https://doi.org/10.1016/j.gaitpost.2004.09.009

Y. Akao, G.H. Mazur, The leading edge in QFD: past, present and future. Int. J. Qual. Reliab. Manag. **20**(1), 20–35 (2003). https://doi.org/10.1108/02656710310453791

"Biomechanics and Motor Control of Human Movement, 4th Edition|Wiley," Wiley.com. Accessed 15 Nov 2021. [Online]. Available: https://www.wiley.com/en-us/Biomechanics+and+Motor+Control+of+Human+Movement%2C+4th+Edition-p-9780470398180

C.A. Davie, A review of Parkinson's disease. Br. Med. Bull. **86**(1), 109–127 (2008). https://doi.org/10.1093/bmb/ldn013

B. Galna, A.T. Murphy, M.E. Morris, Obstacle crossing in Parkinson's disease: mediolateral sway of the centre of mass during level-ground walking and obstacle crossing. Gait Posture **38**(4), 790–794 (2013). https://doi.org/10.1016/j.gaitpost.2013.03.024

H.R. Gonçalves, A.M. Rodrigues, C.P. Santos, Vibrotactile biofeedback devices in Parkinson's disease: a narrative review. Med. Biol. Eng. Comput. **59**(6), 1185–1199 (2021). https://doi.org/10.1007/s11517-021-02365-3

S. Imbesi, G. Mincolelli, Design of smart devices for older people: a user centered approach for the collection of users' needs, in *Intelligent Human Systems Integration 2020*, ed. by T. Ahram, W. Karwowski, A. Vergnano, F. Leali, R. Taiar, in Advances in Intelligent Systems and Computing (Cham: Springer International Publishing, 2020), pp. 860–864. https://doi.org/10.1007/978-3-030-39512-4_131

S. Imbesi, S. Scataglini, A user centered methodology for the design of smart apparel for older users. Sensors **21**(8), Art. no. 8 (2021). https://doi.org/10.3390/s21082804

S. Imbesi, M. Corzani, F. Petrocchi, G. Lopane, L. Chiari, G. Mincolelli, User-centered design of cues with smart glasses for gait rehabilitation in people with Parkinson's disease: a methodology for the analysis of human requirements and cues effectiveness, in *Advances in Simulation and Digital Human Modeling*, ed. by J.L. Wright, D. Barber, S. Scataglini, and S.L. Rajulu, in Lecture Notes in Networks and Systems (Cham: Springer International Publishing, 2021a), pp. 348–358. https://doi.org/10.1007/978-3-030-79763-8_42

S. Imbesi, G. Mincolelli, F. Petrocchi, How to enhance aging people's wellness by means of human centered and co-design methodology, in *Advances in Simulation and Digital Human Modeling*, ed. by D.N. Cassenti, S. Scataglini, S.L. Rajulu, J.L. Wright, in Advances in Intelligent Systems and Computing (Cham: Springer International Publishing, 2021b), pp. 216–225. https://doi.org/10.1007/978-3-030-51064-0_28

S. Imbesi, M. Corzani, G. Lopane, G. Mincolelli, L. Chiari, User-centered design methodologies for the prototype development of a smart harness and related system to provide haptic cues to persons with Parkinson's disease. Sensors **22**(21), Art. no. 21 (2022). https://doi.org/10.3390/s22218095

A.D. Kuo, J.M. Donelan, Dynamic principles of gait and their clinical implications. Phys. Ther. **90**(2), 157–174 (2010). https://doi.org/10.2522/ptj.20090125

B.-C. Lee, A. Fung, T.A. Thrasher, The effects of coding schemes on vibrotactile biofeedback for dynamic balance training in Parkinson's disease and healthy elderly individuals. IEEE Trans. Neural Syst. Rehabil. Eng. **26**(1), 153–160 (2018). https://doi.org/10.1109/TNSRE.2017.2762239

M. Mancini, P. Carlson-Kuhta, C. Zampieri, J.G. Nutt, L. Chiari, F.B. Horak, Postural sway as a marker of progression in Parkinson's disease: a pilot longitudinal study. Gait Posture **36**(3), 471–476 (2012). https://doi.org/10.1016/j.gaitpost.2012.04.010

G. Mincolelli, M. Marchi, S. Imbesi, Inclusive design for ageing people and the internet of things: understanding needs, in *Advances in Design for Inclusion*, ed. by G. Di Bucchianico, P.F. Kercher, in Advances in Intelligent Systems and Computing (Cham: Springer International Publishing, 2018), pp. 98–108. https://doi.org/10.1007/978-3-319-60597-5_9

G. Mincolelli, S. Imbesi, M. Zallio, Collaborative quality function deployment. A methodology for enabling co-design research practice, in *Advances in Design for Inclusion*, ed. by G. Di Bucchianico, in Advances in Intelligent Systems and Computing (Cham: Springer International Publishing, 2020a), pp. 91–99. https://doi.org/10.1007/978-3-030-20444-0_9

G. Mincolelli, G.A. Giacobone, M. Marchi, S. Imbesi, New collaborative version of the quality function deployment: practical application to the HABITAT project, in *Intelligent Human Systems Integration 2020*, ed. by T. Ahram, W. Karwowski, A. Vergnano, F. Leali, R. Taiar, in Advances in Intelligent Systems and Computing (Cham: Springer International Publishing, 2020b), pp. 823–828. https://doi.org/10.1007/978-3-030-39512-4_125

A. Nieuwboer, Cueing for freezing of gait in patients with Parkinson's disease: a rehabilitation perspective. Mov. Disord. off. J. Mov. Disord. Soc. **23**(Suppl 2), S475-481 (2008). https://doi.org/10.1002/mds.21978

D.S. Peterson, F.B. Horak, Neural control of walking in people with parkinsonism. Physiol. Bethesda Md. **31**(2), 95–107 (2016). https://doi.org/10.1152/physiol.00034.2015

A.S. Pollock, B.R. Durward, P.J. Rowe, J.P. Paul, What is balance? Clin. Rehabil. **14**(4), 402–406 (2000). https://doi.org/10.1191/0269215500cr342oa

S.G. Reich, J.M. Savitt, Parkinson's disease. Med. Clin. North Am. **103**(2), 337–350 (2019). https://doi.org/10.1016/j.mcna.2018.10.014

M.W. Rogers, M.-L. Mille, Lateral stability and falls in older people. Exerc. Sport

Sci. Rev. **31**(4), 182–187 (2003). https://doi.org/10.1097/00003677-200310000-00005

M. Schieppati, A. Nardone, Free and supported stance in Parkinson's disease. The effect of posture and 'postural set' on leg muscle responses to perturbation, and its relation to the severity of the disease. Brain J. Neurol. **114**(Pt 3), 1227–1244 (1991). https://doi.org/10.1093/brain/114.3.1227

E.L. Stegemöller, T.A. Buckley, C. Pitsikoulis, E. Barthelemy, R. Roemmich, C.J. Hass, Postural instability and gait impairment during obstacle crossing in Parkinson's disease. Arch. Phys. Med. Rehabil. **93**(4), 703–709 (2012). https://doi.org/10.1016/j.apmr.2011.11.004

M.H. Woollacott, S. Moore, M.H. Hu, Improvements in balance in the elderly through training in sensory organization abilities, in *Sensorimotor impairment in the elderly* (Springer, 1993), pp. 377–392.

M. Zairi, M.A. Youssef, Quality function deployment: a main pillar for successful total quality management and product development. Int. J. Qual. Reliab. Manag. **12**(6), 9–23 (1995). https://doi.org/10.1108/02656719510089894

Cycle 3: System Interface

8

Abstract

The PASSO research project is composed of three design cycles, this chapter presents the third and last cycle aiming to design the graphical interface for the developed system. As in the previous cycles, even the current one was divided into the four phases of planning, analyzing, creating, and verifying. This chapter describes the design process leading to the design of a web app managing the rehabilitation system, and the User-Centered methodology applied to define the users' requirements adopted to guarantee a high level of usability. The designed web app is developed in two main versions: the one for the person affected by Parkinson's disease, which requires a little information and a visualization of the system's feedback, and a version conceived for the medical operator, presenting more options and communicating technical information and parameters about the patient.

8.1 Structure of Cycle 3

The third and last design cycle of the PASSO project aimed to design the graphical interface of the application submitting sensory cues to the user with Parkinson's disease (PD), while practicing the training with the help of the system (Fig. 8.1). It also evaluated the opportunity to design specific interfaces for other categories of users involved in the process. Specifically, in this cycle, the application that manages the system.

The main research questions considered in this final design cycle were: How many users should have a dedicated system interface? Which information and functionalities should have the interface? How should it graphically appear?

During the previous cycles, different sensory cues and the smart wearable devices transmitting them were tested. The whole developed system was composed of feedback, devices, and an app, each corresponding to a design cycle.

During testing protocols, personalization had a very relevant impact on performance effectiveness. Considering cues, some users could follow better auditory cues, differently from others choosing the visual ones. Each person has a peculiar sensitivity to a specific sensory channel that allows them to interpret better signals transmitted to that sense.

Consistently, even in the second design cycle, it was noticed how the possibility of personalization influences the physical, functional, and emotional perception of tested devices.

The use of Co-Design and the application of the QFD tool gave significant results in both previous cycles, and they were used even in the current one.

S. Imbesi, *Inclusive Design of a Smart Device for People with Parkinson's Disease*, Design For Inclusion 4, https://doi.org/10.1007/978-3-031-58249-3_8

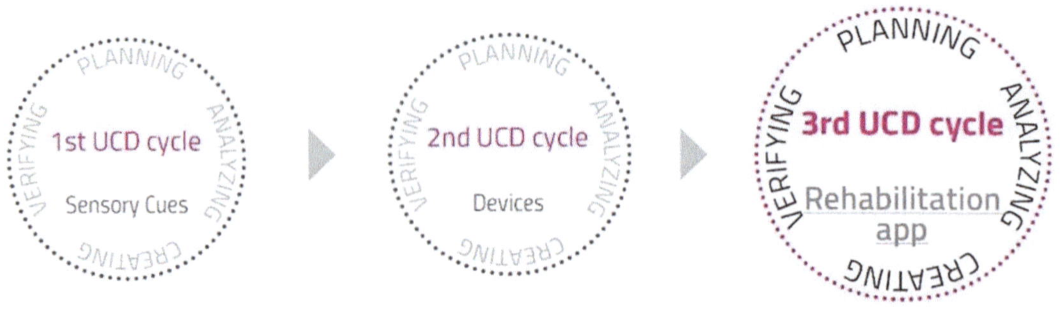

Fig. 8.1 Schematization of the user-centered iterative design cycles

8.2 Planning Phase (C3P1)

After designing cues and devices, this final cycle faced the development of the system app for different users. As seen before, even in this cycle personalization was supposed to be an element significantly impacting the system's usability, for this reason, it was chosen to approach the possibility of developing different interfaces for different users and, for each typology of user, several possibilities of configuration.

This cycle aimed to design and test the application controlling the rehabilitation system to complete the project coherently with the previous stages.

The system under development was conceived to be also used autonomously by patients in their environment, without the assistance of a medical operator, to train themselves.

This design cycle used the same group of interdisciplinary competencies of the past cycles. Indeed, the included professionalisms were:

- Designers (user research, usability, UCD methodology, interaction design, product design, visual design, etc.);
- Technical operators (biomedical engineering, computer science and technology, informatics, etc.);
- Medical operators (neurology, physiatry, physiotherapy, geriatrics, etc.).

Also considered users were the same in the past cycles: person with PD, medical operator, and technical operator.

Understanding the Context

As said in the previous parts of the research project, motor training and gait and posture rehabilitation are fundamental for people with PD to overcome or postpone motor decline characterizing this disease (Peterson and Horak 2016). Beyond aspects strictly related to real-time performance, performance monitoring can make an important contribution to the personalization of the training and the monitoring of impairment evolution. The data collection about the person's walk performance and the elaboration and comparison over time allow monitoring of the person's capabilities and a tailored rehabilitation protocol elaboration.

Symptoms of PD can have wide modifications, changing from the initial to the advanced phases of the disease depending on the individual characteristics and daily lifestyle of the considered person. Motor symptoms such as tremors or movement slowness are the most common during the disease prosecution (Massano and Bhatia 2012).

The progression of motor impairments affects different aspects of daily activities, including the interaction with smartphones. Specifically, tremors and fine motor skills degeneration can invalidate the users' capabilities in handling a smartphone (McNaney et al. 2014).

8.3 Analyzing Phase (C3P2)

For the design of an interface for PD users, the author analyzed which motor, cognitive, and general characteristics affect the interaction between the person and the smartphone (Nunes et al. 2016), and which were the necessities for the categories of users considered in this cycle of the PASSO project.

Some studies documented the difficulties of people with PD using touch screens, observing a 15% error rate in target selection and the variance of touch accuracy during several trials (Montague et al. 2014). For these reasons, it would be desirable to use large targets in screen interfaces to overcome problems related to the weakening of sight and fine motor skills. Moreover, it is useful to design visual elements highly contrasting to ease applications' use (Maziewski et al. 2009).

Besides, considering a large number of studies about touch screen interaction of people with upper limb motor impairments, many of them reported a reduced accuracy in performing tap and swipe gestures (Trewin et al. 2013). To overcome difficulties related to tap kiosk interfaces, it was observed that an enlargement of targets to 20 mm could avoid most of the selection problems (Duff et al. 2010). The enlargement of the tap target proved to be a good strategy even to avoid difficulties brought on by hand tremors (Fisk et al. 2014).

Motor and Cognitive Impairments and General Issues Related to PD

Motor impairments represent the most common and significant PD symptoms, bringing problems affecting autonomy and daily activities.

Bradykinesia causes slowness and a loss of width in repetitive movements. This effect can occur in both gross and fine motor movements. For example, a button selection several consecutive times could become slow and imprecise. Rigidity affects the precision and accuracy of interaction, and the difficulty in moving muscles impacts speed and dexterity in regular tasks. Dyskinesias comes from the excess of medication in the patient's body. It brings uncontrollable involuntary movements that don't allow the person to use a touchscreen easily (Massano and Bhatia 2012).

Tremors caused by PD usually do not significantly impact interaction because they tend to disappear when voluntary movements start (Nunes et al. 2016).

PD sometimes hampers the person's speech, affecting the muscles responsible for this activity. This impairment could compromise the use of natural language for speech interfaces.

Like speech, even the view is sometimes affected by involuntary movements caused by PD. Visual disabilities like blurred and double vision or lower ability to discriminate color and contrast are typical of PD (and of aging).

Another aspect needing attention is that PD decreases the ability to practice multitasking activities. For a PD person, it could be dangerous to interact with a screen if not sitting or standing, avoiding the risk of losing balance. In light of these considerations, an application conceived for this kind of people should not require instant responses from the user.

In PD, cognitive impairments are not as impacting as motor ones but need consideration while designing an interface addressed to users with PD. Usually, PD people are affected by short memory loss, common even to age-related changes, frequently occurring when planning tasks. Together with short memory loss, also thought is affected by PD becoming slower.

Some persons with PD experience depression and apathy even before the onset of motor symptoms. This aspect could result from low motivation in the adaptation to new technologies or frustration in facing new typologies of daily tasks.

Another visible symptom in the advanced stages of PD, as in aging, is cognitive degradation related to a dementia form. This situation is common to almost 15% of the PD population.

PD symptoms present a significant variability in the personal disease evolution and between different people affected by the same disease. This unpredictable evolution makes it difficult to classify users just considering their current PD stage, highlighting a high necessity for tailored solutions based on specific user impairments.

Moreover, considering the single user, it is important to focus on the differences in symptoms between the on and off phases typical of PD, alternating phases of good energy and clarity with phases of weakness and stasis (Davie 2008). Probably, it would be desirable to profile the person in both conditions to provide a specific interaction depending on the current status.

The different progression of PD in every person makes it complicated to find a specific symptom evolution pattern, but the disease seems to be faster in people being affected by the disease in old age. Solutions for PD patients should be adaptable over time to a progressive loss of ability in performing tasks, sometimes in a short period.

Since the beginning of PD impairments, the person experiences a progressive loss of abilities and independence that should be supported by smart systems and interfaces facilitating the maintenance of autonomy.

Selection of Users' Needs

The medical operator of the Istituto di Scienze Neurologiche di Bologna (ISBN) engaged some patients to participate in the project.

All users involved in interviews already had experience in rehabilitation systems for gait and posture training associated with a web application. The following section describes a sample of the nine involved users.

PD Patient 1

She is a young grandmother with a smartphone but uses only basic functions. She feels uncomfortable with new technologies but has an enthusiastic approach to devices supporting her in preserving autonomy and independence.

She tried a rehabilitation system before and commented that sometimes she felt overwhelmed by functions and instructions that she could not manage, but did not stop her sessions with the system. She is not very interested in data but likes to have immediate and simple feedback about the quality of her performances.

Table 8.1 Needs expressed by PD Patient 1

US01	I want to have only the information I need
US02	I want to easily find the functions I need
US03	I want to understand functions clearly
US04	I want to be able to easily read all written parts
US05	I want to know immediately about my performance
US06	I want my parents to be involved in my rehabilitating walks
US07	I want my doctor to be proud of me

She needs to be comforted by the medical operator, and feel a constant connection with him (Table 8.1).

PD Patient 2

He is an engineer, he feels comfortable using smart devices and is not frustrated at all in learning to use new technologies. He is a sporty man and likes to study his performances by analyzing related data. When he is in the On phase, his gait and posture are almost perfect.

He uses other apps to collect different typologies of data about himself and compares results to stimulate himself in increasing his abilities contrasting PD symptoms (Table 8.2).

Medical Operator

She is a physiatrist working on PD and practicing rehabilitation programs for her patients. She likes to experiment with new solutions and devices with her patients, and she is already using smart systems with her patients to monitor their gait and posture.

She appreciates the possibility of collecting gait and posture data to compare them to evaluate the persons' performances over time. In particular, in addition to the parameters collected in cycles 1 and 2, she would like to know how many corrections the system submitted to the

Table 8.2 Needs expressed by PD Patient 2

US08	I want to use it easily even when I am in the Off-phase
US09	I want to press buttons without difficulties
US10	I want to have the possibility to implement functions
US11	I want it to be usable in association with my other devices
US12	I want to compare my performances over time
US13	I want to use it not only for the walk but even for sports like running and climbing
US14	I want to use it even if I have some sight issues

Table 8.3 Needs expressed by the Medical operator

MO01	I want to feel comfortable with the designed digital environment
MO02	I don't want to feel confused about possible functions
MO03	I want to manage the app by myself without the technical operator
MO04	I don't want to see too much information in the app
MO05	I don't want to see information not useful to me
MO06	I want to easily access to parameters I need to know
MO07	I want to match the data collected by the system with the one collected by my traditional tests and protocols
MO08	I want to have more information about the patient's heart rate
MO09	I want to have a report about the single patient's rehabilitation session
MO10	I want to have a report comparing the patient's performance overtime

patient and how many times he was able to correct himself as requested, aiming to establish if self-correction is a viable strategy in the rehabilitation of subjects with PD.

She would also like to have other information about her patient's vital signs like heart rate, pressure, compensatory rate, and compensatory rate variability, that would give her significant information about the user's stress and the disease evolution.

She uses other applications to manage rehabilitation systems but observed a lack of attention in the interface design intended for the medical operators, who have to learn new ways of interaction and interpretation that often discourage and sometimes invalidate the system use (Table 8.3).

Technical Operator

He is a biomedical engineer, he didn't develop the current version of the mHealth system but he worked on its implementation. He usually meets the medical operator, downloads data collected from patients, analyzes data, and finally meets again with the medical operator to show him the obtained results and help with the interpretation due to the developed analysis.

He has no problems with interfaces because conceived by another technician without special regard for other users' categories' needs (Table 8.4).

Analyzing Technologies for Technical Constraints

In this section are analyzed technical aspects involved in the design of the app interface. From these considerations, the characteristics of the project.

Interface Gestures

Typically, actions requested by the user for the use of an interface are tap, swipe, multiple-tap, and drag (Fig. 8.2). Considering people with PD, some of these actions could be difficult to perform for them. Considering guidelines

Table 8.4 Needs expressed by the Technical operator

TO01	I want other users not to complain to me about the app
TO02	I don't want to meet the MO every time I have to download data
TO03	I want to access data even in remote modality
TO04	I want the MO to interpret autonomously obtained results
TO05	I want the MO to use the app properly
TO06	I want the user to use the app properly
TO07	I want the MO to be more autonomous in the system management
TO08	I want the process to last less time from data collection to results transmission

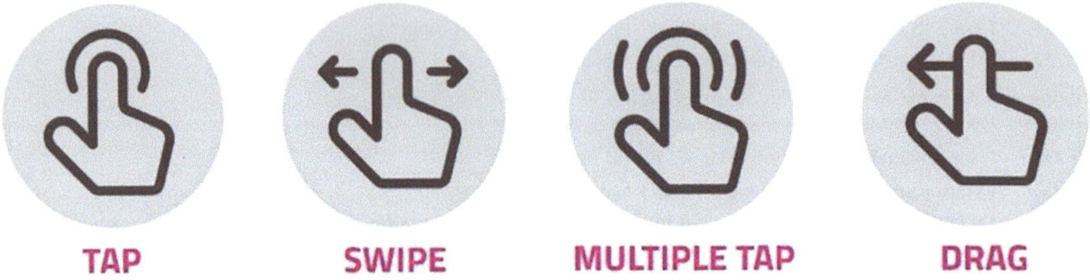

Fig. 8.2 Actions requested by the user for the use of an interface

developed by Nunes et al., some gestures were analyzed (Nunes et al. 2016).

Considering the Tap, when the target size is a square with a side of 14 mm or more, the accuracy level is 97%. If there is not enough space, the target can be reduced to 10,5 mm with a level of accuracy of 94%. The space around the target seems not to influence the accuracy of the single tap, affecting the accuracy level with a 2% decrease.

The swipe gesture usually is not problematic for PD users and there are no significant variations in the performance when the target size changes, or when the distance between the target and its surroundings decreases. Commonly, the swipe movement speed for people with PD is 24 mm/s.

The multiple tap does not bring particular issues in precision and speed until the tenth tap when the user is in the On phase. There are no trials considering users in the Off phase.

The drag gesture is usually performed successfully but with a very slow movement. Users were able to choose one element and drag it, taking 4 s to reach the desired position. Considering actions when it is possible to choose between multiple taps and Drag, PD users seem to prefer the Multiple-tap solution.

Touch Interaction

Considering scientific literature regarding the design of smartphone applications addressed to users with PD, several guidelines have been extrapolated (Nunes et al. 2016).

- Tap targets should have a side size of 14 mm (minimum 10,5 mm, maximum 21 mm), similar to what is recommended for older users (Leitao and Silva 2012). Recommended size allows this category of users to have a performance similar to one of the mainstream users (target side size 7–10 mm) (Park et al. 2008).
- Swipe gesture does not require a specific target size to be performed by people with PD, differently from aging users who prefer wider targets. The only aspect to consider is that PD users commonly swipe at 24 m, so avoiding activation speed would be preferable.

- Multiple taps can be used for controls because they do not create issues until 10 taps. However, this gesture should not be repeated too many consequent times because it could discourage the user.
- Drag gestures should be used sparingly, PD users can do this action successfully but in a very slow way so it could be a little frustrating and compromise the interface comfort level.
- Multiple taps should be used instead of Drag when possible, users can play properly both actions but multiple taps have shown it is more performing.
- A high possibility of adaptation is required for interfaces for users with PD due to the variability of symptoms. An app should be able to detect changes in the user's interaction and modify itself to optimize his/her gestures.

Information Display

After analyzing recommendations regarding gestures, strategies to display information were evaluated.

It would be desirable to use colored and highly contrasting elements, to avoid issues in distinguishing targets. PD can impact sight and compromise the ability to evaluate differences below low contrasts (Nunes et al. 2016).

Considering short-term memory loss, happening both in PD patients and aging users, the amount of information displayed needs to be carefully evaluated in order not to stress the person (Foltynie et al. 2004).

Even slowness of thought and movements can influence the interaction between the person and the smartphone, due to this, time-dependent controls should be avoided to reduce the user's stress and frustration leading him to have an uncomfortable perception of the interface.

Due to impairments affecting speech and vision, it would be desirable to give the possibility of using both channels for interaction, enhancing the applications' usability over time, and considering potential incoming limitations of the user. This strategy is suitable even to overcome issues related to Off phases.

Table 8.5 Table of selected characteristics

C01	Target size (mm)
C02	Space between targets (mm)
C03	Letters dimension (mm)
C04	Maximum number of targets in a screen (n)
C05	Colors' contrast between target and background (△E)
C06	Number of possible gestures (n)
C07	Number of the information displayed per screen (n)
C08	Maximum number of taps to complete a task (n)
C09	Maximum number of visualized screens to complete a task (n)
C10	Number of sensory channels involved in completing a task (n)

Most PD people experience the disease in old age, which is why aging symptoms should always be considered when designing for this category of users (Kurniawan and Zaphiris 2005).

Selected Characteristics

In the following Table 8.5 are listed characteristics extrapolated by scientific literature dedicated to digital interfaces addressed to PD people. The selected characteristics are measurable parameters concerning the structure and graphics of the system app.

8.4 Creating Phase (C3P3)

In the creating phase users were considered separately, and for each one the multidisciplinary team elaborated a Quality Function Deployment matrix, to understand which interface characteristics could mostly influence the usability of the final version of the webapp.

Quality Function Deployment

As in the other cycles, even in this one, the QFD was used for its traditional objective (Zairi and Youssef 1995): users' needs and project's characteristics are reported in the QFD matrix to evaluate their degree of relationship (Mincolelli et al. 2020), and to give different levels of importance to selected characteristics for effective development of the design cycle (Imbesi and Mincolelli 2020).

After selecting the final needs, the team attributed a mark to the degree of relationship between every need and every characteristic.

Those scores were reported in boxes of intersections between lines and columns using the following classification:

- 0 (light gray): The cue does not respond to the need
- 1 (light pink): The cue weakly responds to the need
- 3 (pink): The cue satisfactorily responds to the need
- 9 (magenta): The cue strongly responds to the need

Thus, using these marks, the QFD algorithm elaborated values, expressed in percentage, representing the relative and absolute importance of each characteristic in consideration of the other ones listed in the matrix.

was decided to elaborate on three different QFDs for three different applications, each one dedicated to a category of users involved in the design cycle.

Quality Function Deployment of Users with PD

The first QFD matrix was addressed to PD users (Fig. 8.3). Collected needs were listed, grouping them depending on the argument. Finally, needs were divided into the groups of aesthetics, functions, and emotions.

After completing the QFD matrix with the degree of correlation between the needs and characteristics of the primary users, characteristics were listed following the order of importance resulting from the application of the tool (Table 8.6).

Looking at the table of characteristics importance, it is possible to notice that the first ones refer to aspects related to usability.

The first characteristic is the "Number of information displayed by the system" which helps the user not to feel overwhelmed by the information given by the app. This aspect needs to be balanced with the "maximum number of visualized screens to complete a task" requested to be low for the same reason.

The second characteristic is the "maximum number of targets per screen" which is quite similar to the one before but regards the number of issues to be selectable on the same screen. When there are too many targets, the user could have difficulties in the selection caused of their small dimension or the low space between them.

The third characteristic is "the number of sensory channels involved to complete a task", which could affect or improve the app's usability. Involving more senses could help the patient in the app management, simplifying the interaction, but, depending on the person, it could be also an obstacle if requiring high multitasking abilities that are often compromised in people with PD.

Quality Function Deployment of Medical Operators

The second QFD matrix was addressed to the Modical Operator (Fig. 8.4). Collected needs were listed, dividing them depending on the argument. Finally needs were divided into the groups of aesthetics and functions.

After completing the QFD matrix with the degree of correlation between the needs and characteristics of the primary users, characteristics were listed following the order of importance resulting from the application of the tool (Table 8.7).

Regarding the Medical Operator, the most relevant characteristics refer to the app structure that needs to be easy and quick to use.

The most significant characteristic, such as in the previous table addressed to the user with PD, was the "Number of the information displayed per screen". In this case, it is possible to give more information per screen, paying attention to the selection, to provide all searched information in a few screens easily manageable by the Medical Operator.

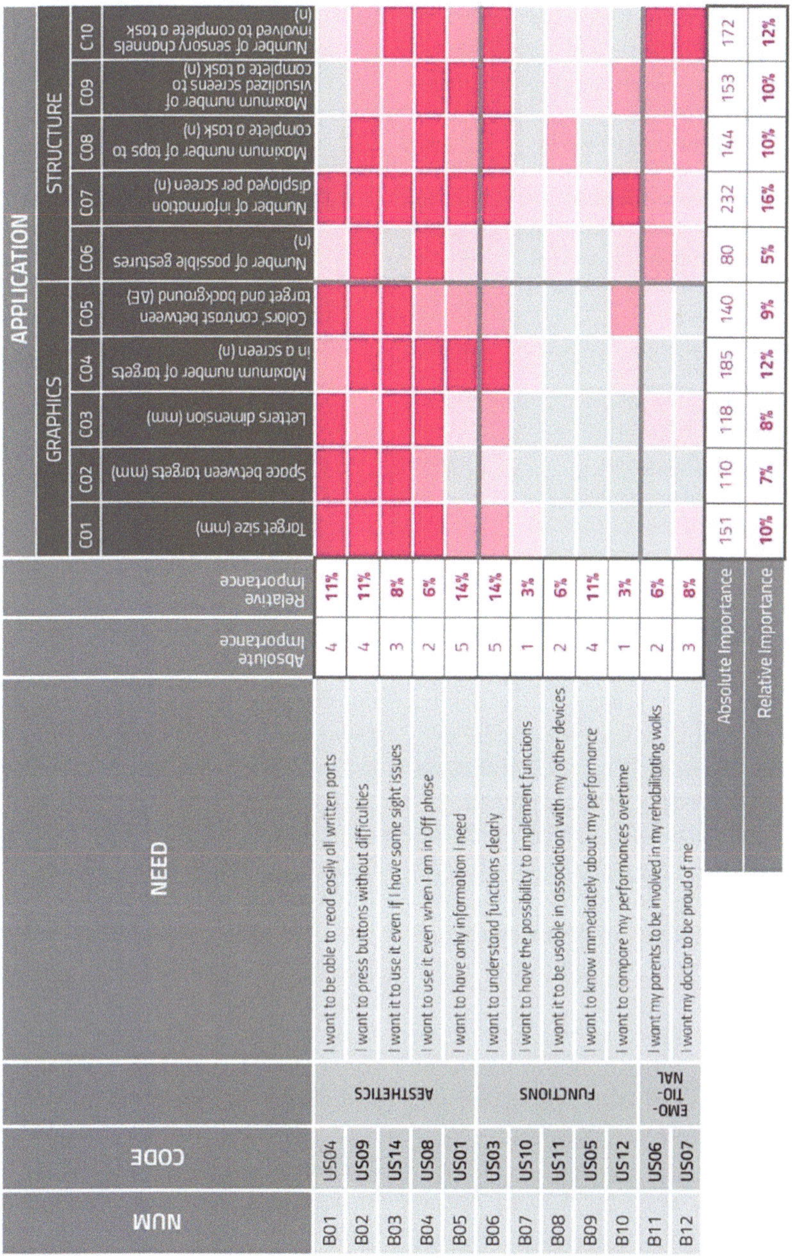

Fig. 8.3 QFD matrix addressed to the PD user

The second characteristic for importance is the "Maximum number of taps to complete a task" which reflects the operator's necessity of spending as little time as possible in setting up and consulting the app, especially when at the same time interacting with the patient with PD.

The third characteristic for importance is the "Maximum number of visualized screens to complete a task", which is related to the previous ones and underlines the necessity for this category of users to be agile in the interaction with the app, not wasting time and not making patients wait and get bored during their medical consultation.

Table 8.6 Table of characteristics importance in relation with PD users

Code	Characteristic	Field	Relative importance	Absolute importance (%)
C07	Number of the information displayed per screen (n)	Structure	232	16
C04	Maximum number of targets in a screen (n)	Graphics	185	12
C10	Number of sensory channels involved in completing a task (n)	Structure	172	12
C09	Maximum number of visualized screens to complete a task (n)	Structure	153	10
C01	Target size (mm)	Graphics	151	10
C08	Maximum number of taps to complete a task (n)	Structure	144	10
C05	Colors' contrast between target and background (△E)	Graphics	140	9
C03	Letters dimension (mm)	Graphics	118	8
C02	Space between targets (mm)	Graphics	110	7
C06	Number of possible gestures (n)	Structure	80	5

Quality Function Deployment of Technical Operators

The third and last QFD matrix was addressed to the Technical Operator (Fig. 8.5). Collected needs were listed depending on the argument.

After completing the QFD matrix with the degree of correlation between the needs and characteristics of the primary users, characteristics were listed again following the new order of importance resulting from the application of the tool (Table 8.8).

Trying to interpret the characteristics' hierarchization emerging from the Technical Operator QFD, it is possible to notice that the most important ones all refer to aspects regarding the app structure.

As for the other users and medical operators, the most significant characteristic was the "Number of information displayed per screen" which surely influences the degree of usability of the app. This parameter is related to the number of actions that are possible to carry out using the app, and to its effectiveness.

The second characteristic was the "Maximum number of visualized screens to complete a task" which is set by the Technical Operator for each typology of user and significantly influences the perception of users about the app's ease of use.

The third characteristic is the "Maximum number of taps to complete a task" that, as previously described for the Medical Operator" allows users to spend only a little time in setting and using the app.

Developing Design and Technological Solutions

Thanks to considerations allowed by QFD matrices, it was designed an app structure for each category of users involved in the project. The following schemes describe the functions desirable to include in the different apps.

Building Prototypes: PD User

As described before, users with PD are very sensitive to interface graphics due to their potential hand-motor impairments. Other problematic elements are functions engaging both multitasking activities and short-term memory. One of the possible strategies to overcome these limitations is the reduction of functions, keeping only the necessary ones, and the deletion of not strictly fundamental information.

This category of users is supposed to use the app when practicing a rehabilitation session by themselves in their environment. They require

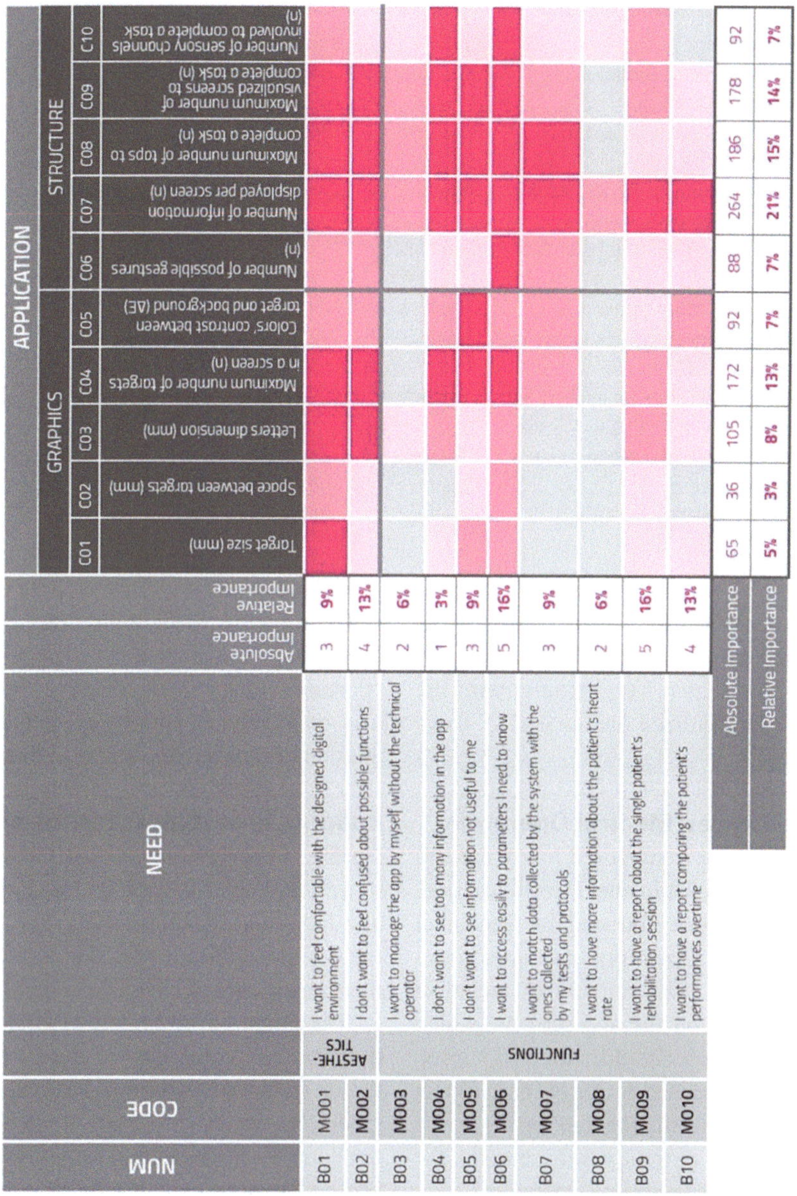

Fig. 8.4 QFD matrix addressed to the Medical Operator

to manage the system comfortably without facing technical issues they cannot fix. At the same time, another fundamental aspect is the gratification they need as encouragement for the training: the system is supposed to give graphic feedback, allowing users to see their performance progress and to have a motivation for their motor improvement (Fig. 8.6).

Fundamental functions were identified in "new training session", starting a new session (following parameters previously set by the Medical Operator), and giving the possibility to have a report about it; "past training sessions" to visualize a comparison of present and past performances;"contact" to transmit an alert about malfunctioning of the system to the Medical

Table 8.7 Table of characteristics importance in relation with Medical Operators

Code	Characteristic	Field	Relative importance	Absolute importance (%)
C07	Number of the information displayed per screen (n)	Structure	264	21
C08	Maximum number of taps to complete a task (n)	Structure	186	15
C09	Maximum number of visualized screens to complete a task (n)	Structure	178	14
C04	Maximum number of targets in a screen (n)	Graphics	172	13
C03	Letters dimension (mm)	Graphics	105	8
C05	Colors' contrast between target and background ($\triangle E$)	Graphics	92	7
C10	Number of sensory channels involved in completing a task (n)	Structure	92	7
C06	Number of possible gestures (n)	Structure	88	7
C01	Target size (mm)	Graphics	65	5
C02	Space between targets (mm)	Graphics	36	3

Operator and, finally, "send data" to send the system collected data for their elaboration.

The app structure was very simple, with the possibility of personalized items not to overwhelm the person.

Building Prototypes: Medical Operator

The Medical Operator is supposed to use the app to register the patient, set his/her thresholds, and, finally, consult results elaborated by Technical Operators. Medical Operators are sometimes overwhelmed by the huge amount of technical information reported on the app screens, which is unnecessary for them and difficult to interpret. This problem is not related to the graphic aspect of communicated information but involves the app structure that is currently substantially the same for Medical and Technical Operators.

Another issue that emerged from interviews is the desire of the Medical Operator to have specific reports of data collected during performances (Fig. 8.7).

Fundamental functions addressed to the Medical Operator are "New patient", giving the possibility to register the user listing relevant clinical data about his pathologies and impairments; "Choose patient", allowing to see previously registered data of the person and reports regarding the single current training and past training sessions, and comparing them with other clinical trends considered significant for the specific person; and "Posture settings" to directly start the training session or to modify parameters related to the submission of sensory cues to the defined patient.

Building Prototypes: Technical Operator

During interviews with Technical Operators, it was registered a lack of needs regarding the app functions for themselves. The reason is that the current interface was conceived considering their needs, which have been satisfied yet.

The attention of Technical Operators goes to the other two categories of users interacting with the system. Considering PD users, Technical Operators want them to be satisfied with the system, and to use it easily without issues creating a sense of frustration and refusal.

On the other hand, considering Medical Operators, Technical Operators need to develop solutions involving them and making them more autonomous in using the system and interpreting its outputs.

Finding effective solutions to reduce the effort of data elaboration and results interpretation up to the Technical Operator, would save a lot of time.

For these reasons, it was decided not to develop a specific app interface for the Technical Operator, but to focus on the other categories of users.

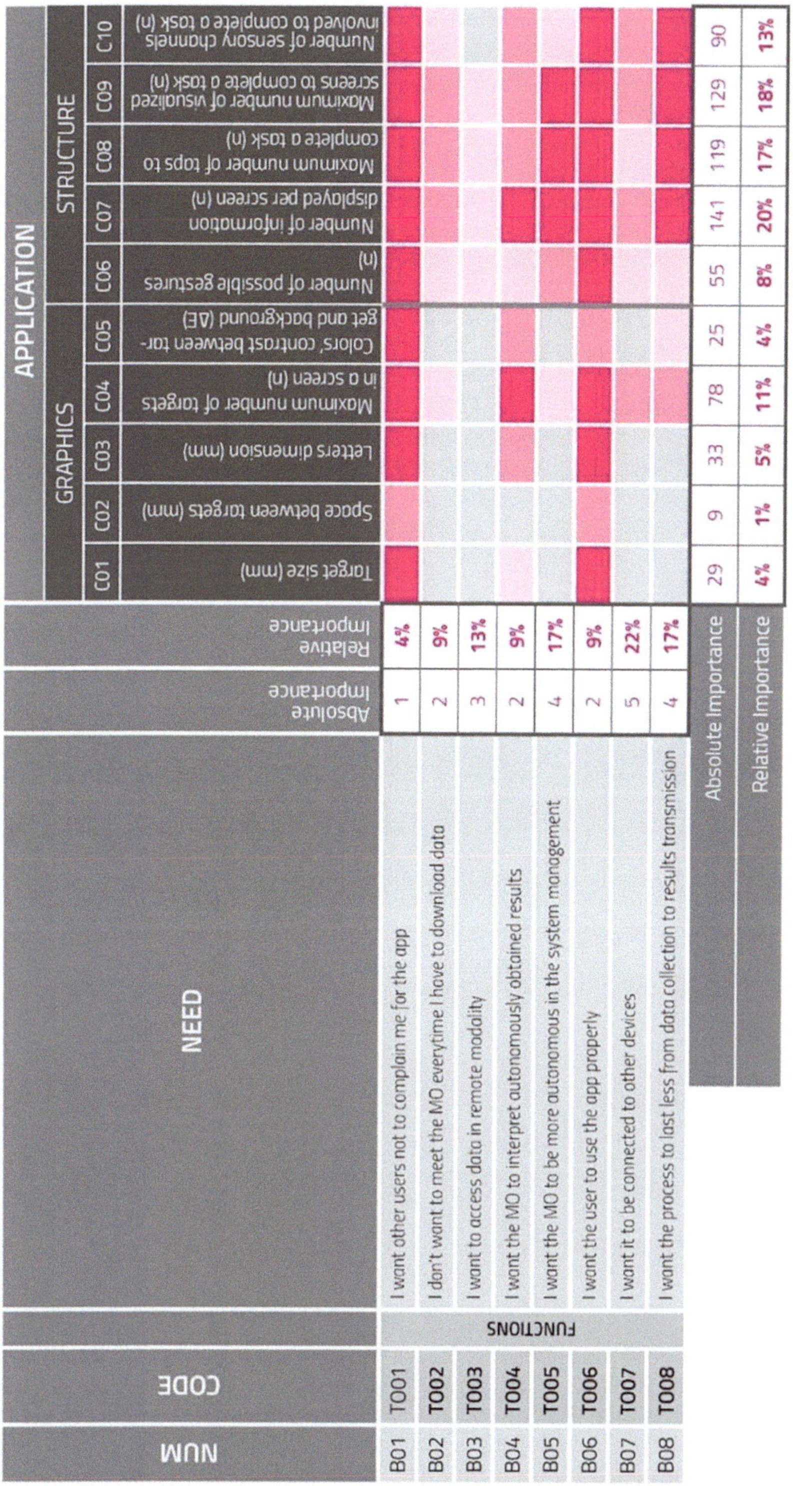

Fig. 8.5 QFD matrix addressed to the Technical Operator

Table 8.8 Table of characteristics importance in relation with Technical Operators

Code	Characteristic	Field	Relative importance	Absolute importance (%)
C07	Number of the information displayed per screen (n)	Structure	141	20
C09	Maximum number of visualized screens to complete a task (n)	Structure	129	18
C08	Maximum number of taps to complete a task (n)	Structure	119	17
C10	Number of sensory channels involved in completing a task (n)	Structure	90	13
C04	Maximum number of targets in a screen (n)	Graphics	78	11
C06	Number of possible gestures (n)	Structure	55	8
C03	Letters dimension (mm)	Graphics	33	5
C01	Target size (mm)	Graphics	29	4
C05	Colors' contrast between target and background ($\triangle$E)	Graphics	25	4
C02	Space between targets (mm)	Graphics	9	1

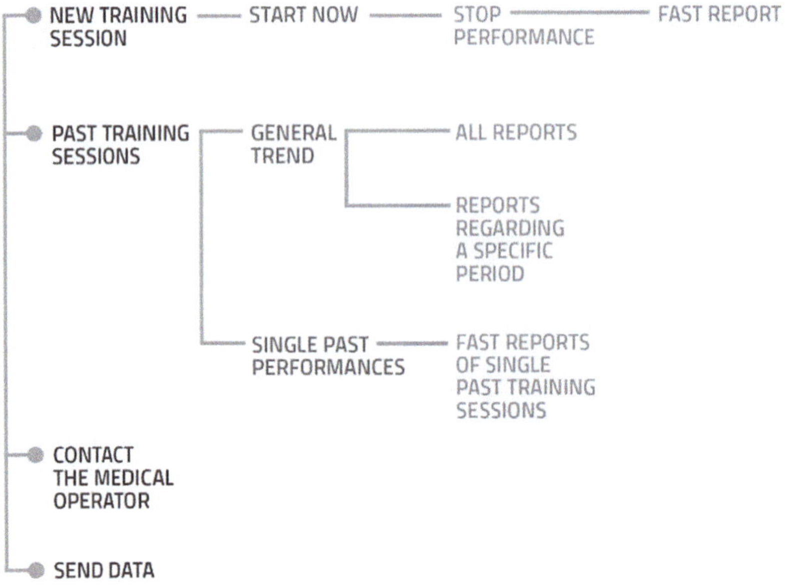

Fig. 8.6 Scheme representing functions for the user with PD for easy system management

8.5 Conclusions

This chapter describes the first three phases of the last design cycle of the PASSO project. In this cycle, the author designed the interface of the smart system submitting vibratory cues to people with PD. After an analysis of technologies and users' capabilities and requirements, the use of the QFD helped to hierarchize called information to obtain a list of the most important graphical interface characteristics about structure and graphics for each category of users (User with PD, Medical Operator, Technical Operator). At this point of the process, the web app managing the system was prototyped in two different versions: one for the PD patient, and the other for the medical operator.

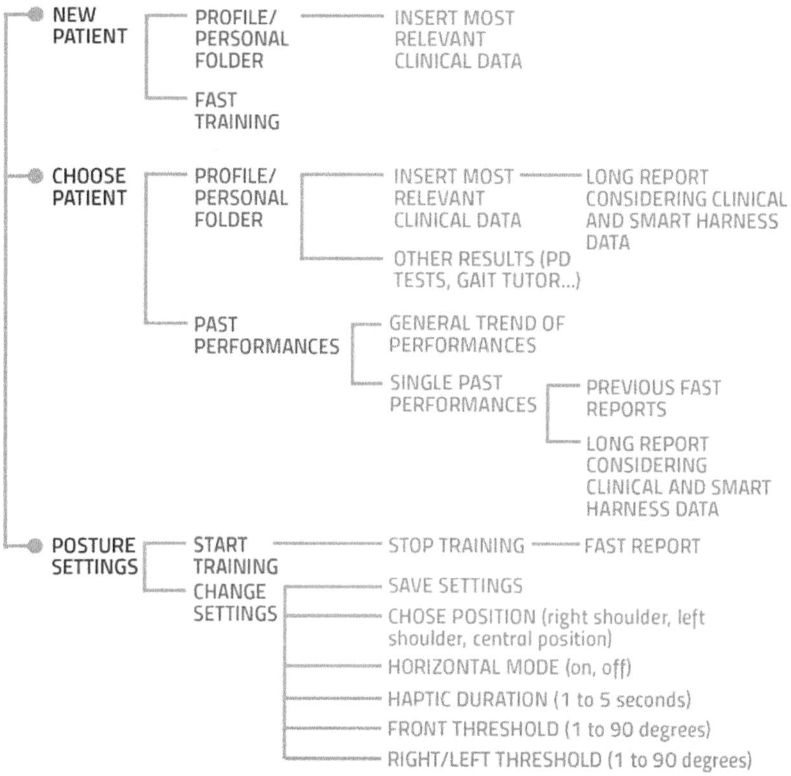

Fig. 8.7 Scheme representing functions useful to the medical operator for easy management of the system

The chosen methodology allowed the multidisciplinary team to collect the most important characteristics of each typology user, whose involvement was fundamental for developing prototypes following a tailored structure satisfying the needs of people involved in the design process.

References

C.A. Davie, A review of Parkinson's disease. Br. Med. Bull. **86**(1), 109–127 (2008). https://doi.org/10.1093/bmb/ldn013

S.N. Duff, C.B. Irwin, J.L. Skye, M.E. Sesto, D.A. Wiegmann, The effect of disability and approach on touch screen performance during a number entry task. Proc. Hum. Factors Ergon. Soc. Annu. Meet. **54**(6), 566–570 (2010). https://doi.org/10.1177/154193121005400605

D. Fisk, N. Charness, S.J. Czaja, W.A. Rogers, J. Sharit, *Designing for Older Adults*. London: CRC Press, (2014). https://doi.org/10.1201/9781482284775

T. Foltynie, C.E.G. Brayne, T.W. Robbins, R.A. Barker, The cognitive ability of an incident cohort of Parkinson's patients in the UK. The CamPaIGN study. Brain **127**(3), 550–560 (2004). https://doi.org/10.1093/brain/awh067

S. Imbesi , G. Mincolelli, Monitoring older people: an overview of devices responding to significant needs of elderly affected by Parkinson's disease, in *Advances in Additive Manufacturing, Modeling Systems and 3D Prototyping*, M. Di Nicolantonio, E. Rossi, and T. Alexander, Eds., in Advances in Intelligent Systems and Computing. Cham: Springer International Publishing, pp. 646–656 (2020). https://doi.org/10.1007/978-3-030-20216-3_60

S. Kurniawan, P. Zaphiris, Research-derived web design guidelines for older people, in *Proceedings of the 7th international ACM SIGACCESS conference on Computers and accessibility*, in Assets '05. New York, NY, USA: Association for Computing Machinery, pp. 129–135 (2005). https://doi.org/10.1145/1090785.1090810.

R. Leitao, P.A. Silva, Target and spacing sizes for smartphone user interfaces for older adults : design patterns based on an evaluation with users, presented at the Conference on Pattern Languages of Programs, Arizona, United States, 2012. Accessed: Oct. 27,

2021. [Online]. Available: http://www.hillside.net/plop/2012/papers/Group%201%20-%20Elk/Target%20and%20Spacing%20Sizes%20for%20Smartphone%20User%20interfaces%20for%20Older%20Adults%20-%20Design%20patterns%20Based%20on%20an%20Evaluation%20with%20Users.pdf!

J. Massano, K.P. Bhatia, Clinical approach to Parkinson's disease: features, diagnosis, and principles of management. Cold Spring Harb. Perspect. Med. **2**(6), a008870 (2012). https://doi.org/10.1101/cshperspect.a008870

P. Maziewski, P. Suchomski, B. Kostek, A. Czyzewski, An intuitive graphical user interface for the Parkinson's Disease patients, in *2009 4th International IEEE/EMBS Conference on Neural Engineering*, pp. 14–17 (2009). https://doi.org/10.1109/NER.2009.5109223

R. McNaney et al., Exploring the acceptability of google glass as an everyday assistive device for people with parkinson's, in *Proceedings of the SIGCHI Conference on Human Factors in Computing Systems*, in CHI '14. New York, NY, USA: Association for Computing Machinery, pp. 2551–2554 (2014). https://doi.org/10.1145/2556288.2557092.

G. Mincolelli, G.A. Giacobone, M. Marchi, S. Imbesi, New collaborative version of the quality function deployment: practical application to the HABITAT project, in *Intelligent Human Systems Integration 2020*, T. Ahram, W. Karwowski, A. Vergnano, F. Leali, and R. Taiar, Eds., in Advances in Intelligent Systems and Computing. Cham: Springer International Publishing, pp. 823–828 (2020). https://doi.org/10.1007/978-3-030-39512-4_125

K. Montague, H. Nicolau, V.L. Hanson, Motor-impaired touchscreen interactions in the wild, in *Proceedings of the 16th international ACM SIGACCESS conference on Computers & accessibility*, in ASSETS '14. New York, NY, USA: Association for Computing Machinery, pp. 123–130 (2014). https://doi.org/10.1145/2661334.2661362

F. Nunes, P.A. Silva, J. Cevada, A. Correia Barros, L. Teixeira, User interface design guidelines for smartphone applications for people with Parkinson's disease, Univers. Access Inf. Soc. **15**(4), 659–679 (2016). https://doi.org/10.1007/s10209-015-0440-1

Y.S. Park, S.H. Han, J. Park, Y. Cho, Touch key design for target selection on a mobile phone, in *Proceedings of the 10th international conference on Human computer interaction with mobile devices and services*, in MobileHCI '08. New York, NY, USA: Association for Computing Machinery, pp. 423–426 (2008). https://doi.org/10.1145/1409240.1409304

D.S. Peterson, F.B. Horak, Neural control of walking in people with Parkinsonism. Physiol. Bethesda Md. **31**(2), 95–107 (2016). https://doi.org/10.1152/physiol.00034.2015

S. Trewin, C. Swart, D. Pettick, Physical accessibility of touchscreen smartphones, in *Proceedings of the 15th International ACM SIGACCESS Conference on Computers and Accessibility*, in ASSETS '13. New York, NY, USA: Association for Computing Machinery, pp. 1–8 (2013). https://doi.org/10.1145/2513383.2513446.

M. Zairi, M.A. Youssef, Quality function deployment: a main pillar for successful total quality management and product development. Int. J. Qual. Reliab. Manag. **12**(6), 9–23 (1995). https://doi.org/10.1108/02656719510089894

9 Cycle 3: Verifying Phase

Abstract

This chapter describes the last part of the design process of the project of the interface of a web app managing the smart system submitting haptic feedback to train the gait and posture of people affected by Parkinson's Disease. During this last part of the cycle, the multidisciplinary research team involved in the project, together with representatives of the selected category of users, developed the prototypes of a web app submitting the sensory cues. The app prototypes are structured following the requirements of the two main typologies of users using them: patients with Parkinson's disease training themselves to improve their gait and posture to slow their motor degeneration; and medical operators rehabilitating patients with gait and posture impairments by planning, setting, and collecting data about their training session enhanced by the application of smart systems.

9.1 Web App Prototypes

The design of the smart system interface rehabilitating the gait and posture of people affected by Parkinson's disease (PD) requires a high degree of usability for each different category of users considered as related to the use of the project's outcomes (Johnson and Finn 2017; Nunes et al. 2016).

In the previous chapter, the author described the first part of this third design cycle where the planning, analyzing, and creating User-Centered phases led to the structure of prototypes addressed to patients with Parkinson's Disease (PD) and medical operators taking care of them. The current chapter describes the final verifying phase of the third project cycle, showing the designed prototypes then tested with the users' representatives involved in the project's process.

An app mockup was developed to test user interactions and the interface. Prototyping aimed to create an interface for the user with PD and one for the Medical Operator.

Regarding primary users, the focus was on reducing information and functions to simplify the use for people with motor, sight, and cognitive impairments. Written parts were reduced, targets were enlarged and dimensions and contrasts between different elements were used to create a visual hierarchy of the targets on every screen (Young et al. 2017; Maziewski et al. 2009).

Contrariwise, for Medical Operators the developed app structure, had the objective of simplifying functions and data sharing with Medical Operators.

In the following pages are reported some screens of both developed app interfaces developed in the Italian language due to the necessity of testing with Italian users.

The user's interface was developed to be used on his own in his house or where he/she decides

S. Imbesi, *Inclusive Design of a Smart Device for People with Parkinson's Disease*, Design For Inclusion 4, https://doi.org/10.1007/978-3-031-58249-3_9

to practice the training session. The medical operator's interface was developed to be used in the ambulatory context while setting the personalized training program (Fig. 9.1).

App Interface for Users with PD

The users' app has only the fundamental functions. It is developed to have wide buttons and reduced cognitive effort. It is developed to be used intuitively by the person on his/her own.

On the first screen, the user can choose one of the three main functions (Fig. 9.2).

When the user selects "New session", he can see this screen to begin the training (Fig. 9.3).

When the user selects "Start", he is led to the page of the single training, visualizing passed time and allowing the stop of the session (Fig. 9.4).

When the user selects "Stop of the training", he can see this screen visualizing the most important information and parameters collected during the training session (Fig. 9.5).

Moreover, for the user is possible to visualize the old sessions and have information about them to make comparisons with other training sessions (Fig. 9.6).

The section "Instruction" presents some pictures and sentences about how to wear the smart harness (Fig. 9.7).

The user can use the "Help" function to make a call with the medical operator to ask questions about the app or to report a malfunction (Fig. 9.8).

App Interface for Medical Operator

The medical operator's interface needed to be easy and quick to use, following the necessities of medical operators' collected needs.

The app allows the choice of registered patients and the creation of new patient profiles (Fig. 9.9).

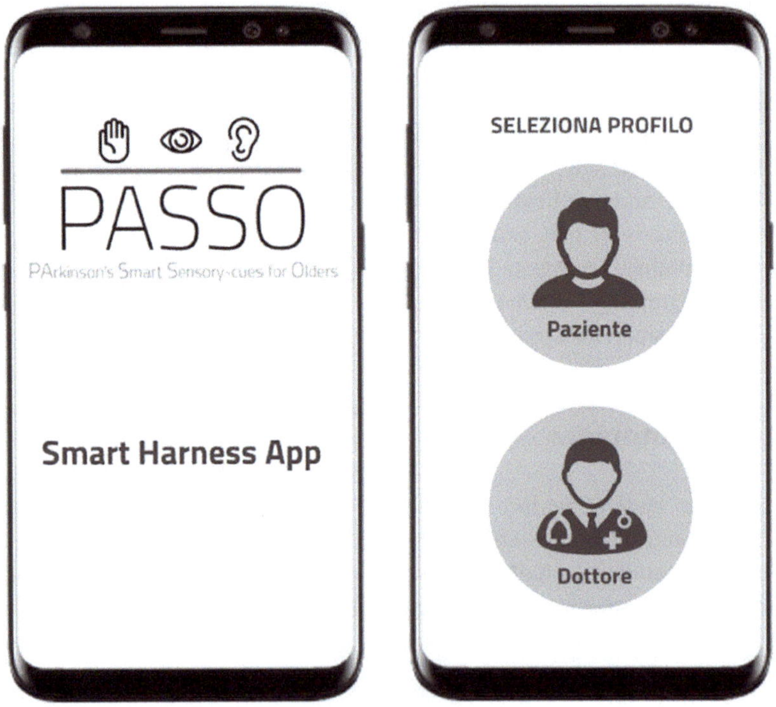

Fig. 9.1 The first screens allow the selection of the users' profiles

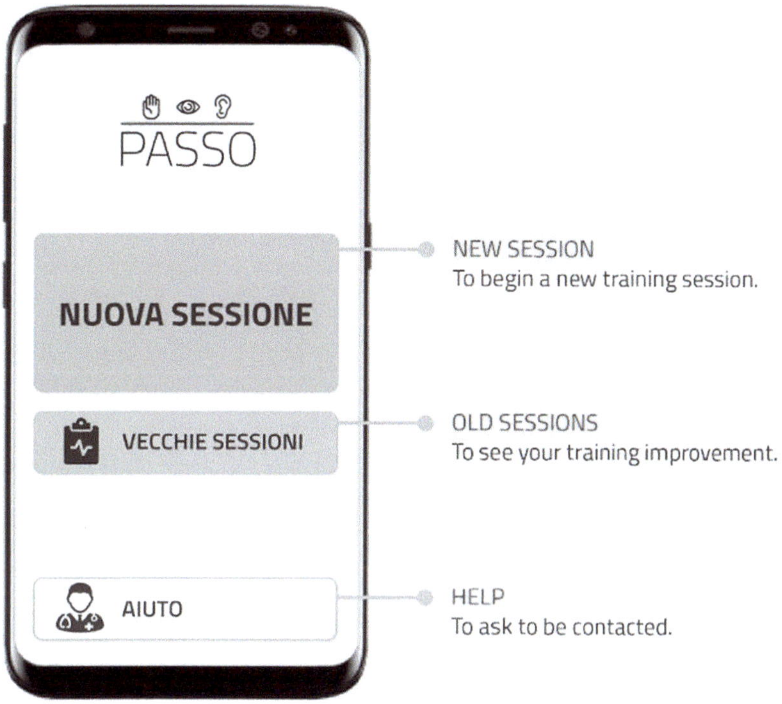

Fig. 9.2 First screen in user modality

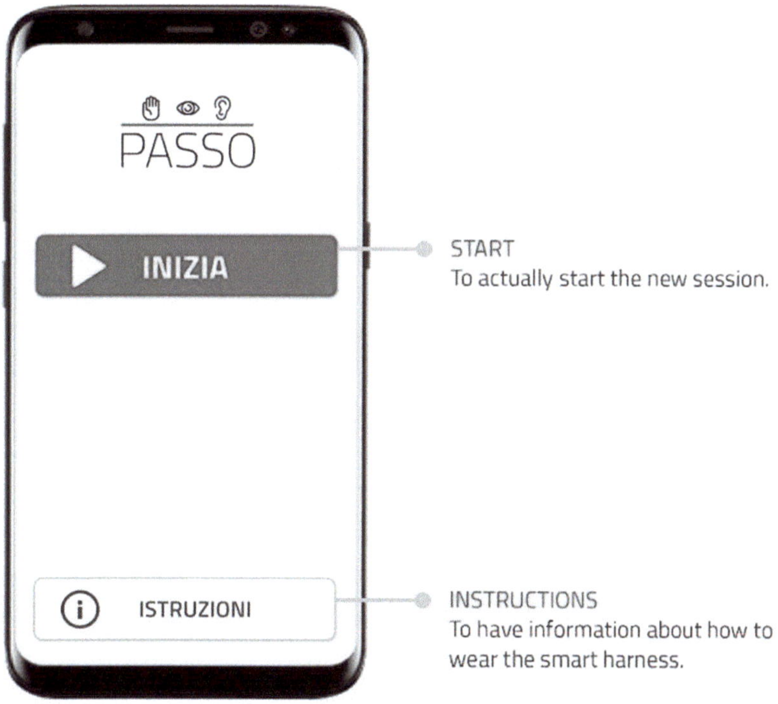

Fig. 9.3 Screen of the beginning session

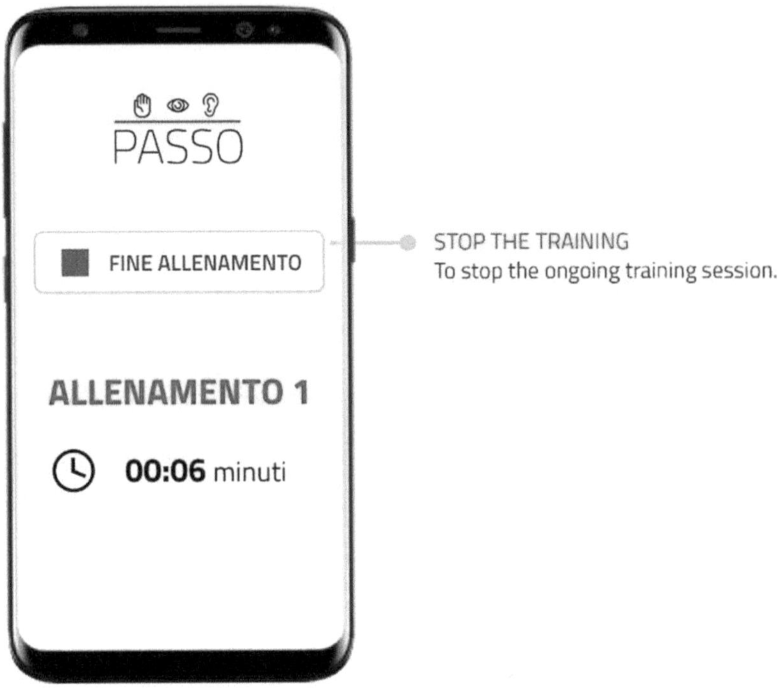

Fig. 9.4 Screen that the user sees during his/her training session

Fig. 9.5 Screen of the training session report for the PD user

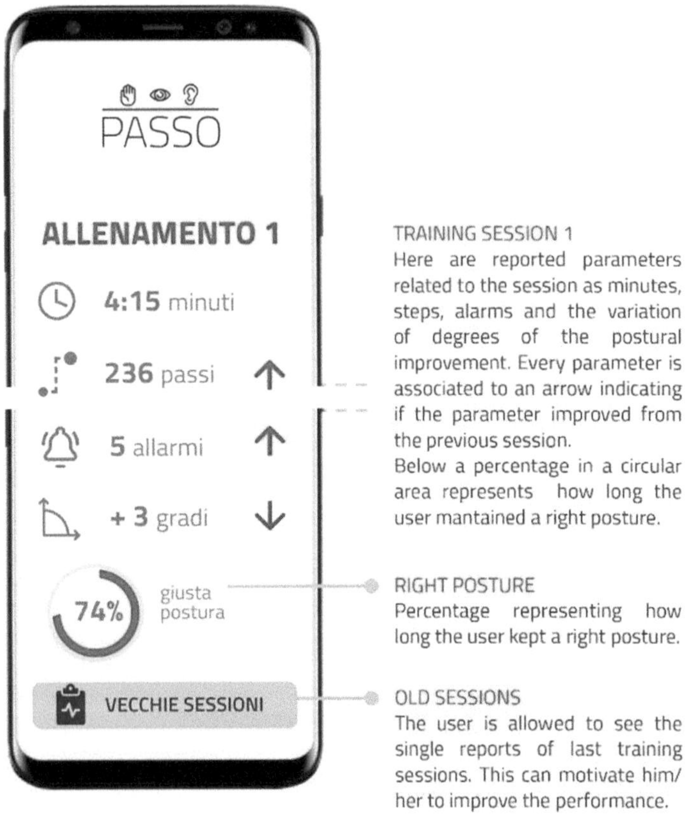

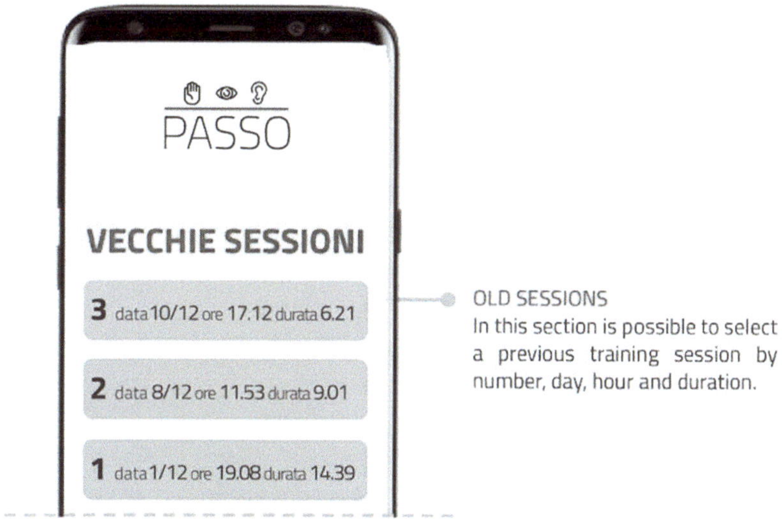

Fig. 9.6 Screen collecting old training session reports

After choosing the patient, the Medical Operator can fill or modify the related information.

The first view is about the patient's profile (Fig. 9.10).

The second icon of the Medical Operator's interface leads to the "Settings" menu (Fig. 9.11).

The third icon of the Medical Operator's interface leads to the "Old Sessions" menu (Fig. 9.12).

The last icon of the Medical Operator's interface allows the beginning of the current training session (Fig. 9.13).

The final report of the training session shows the Medical Operator several parameters that can be collected for a long-term evaluation (Fig. 9.14).

9.2 Testing with Users

The testing protocol was divided into several phases, everyone aiming to test several functions for PD users and Medical Operators. In each phase, it was given a task to be completed, and it evaluated several aspects related to the quality of the interaction.

Medical and Technical Operators testing the app were informally questioned about their impressions of the ease of use, accessibility, effectiveness, usability, and usefulness of the tested interfaces.

Testing Protocol for Users with PD

Regarding PD users, inclusion and exclusion criteria comprised the diagnosis of Medical Operators, and Technical Operators participating in this testing phase were the ones involved in the previous stages of the design process.

The testing protocol was applied in an ambulatory context informally.

The equipment consisted of a smartphone where the app mockup containing both patient and doctor profiles was installed.

The Operators were asked to carry out some tasks as patients:

- Access your profile
- Find instructions about wearing the smart harness
- Ask for help from your doctor
- Look at your past performances
- Start a new training session
- Look at your training session report

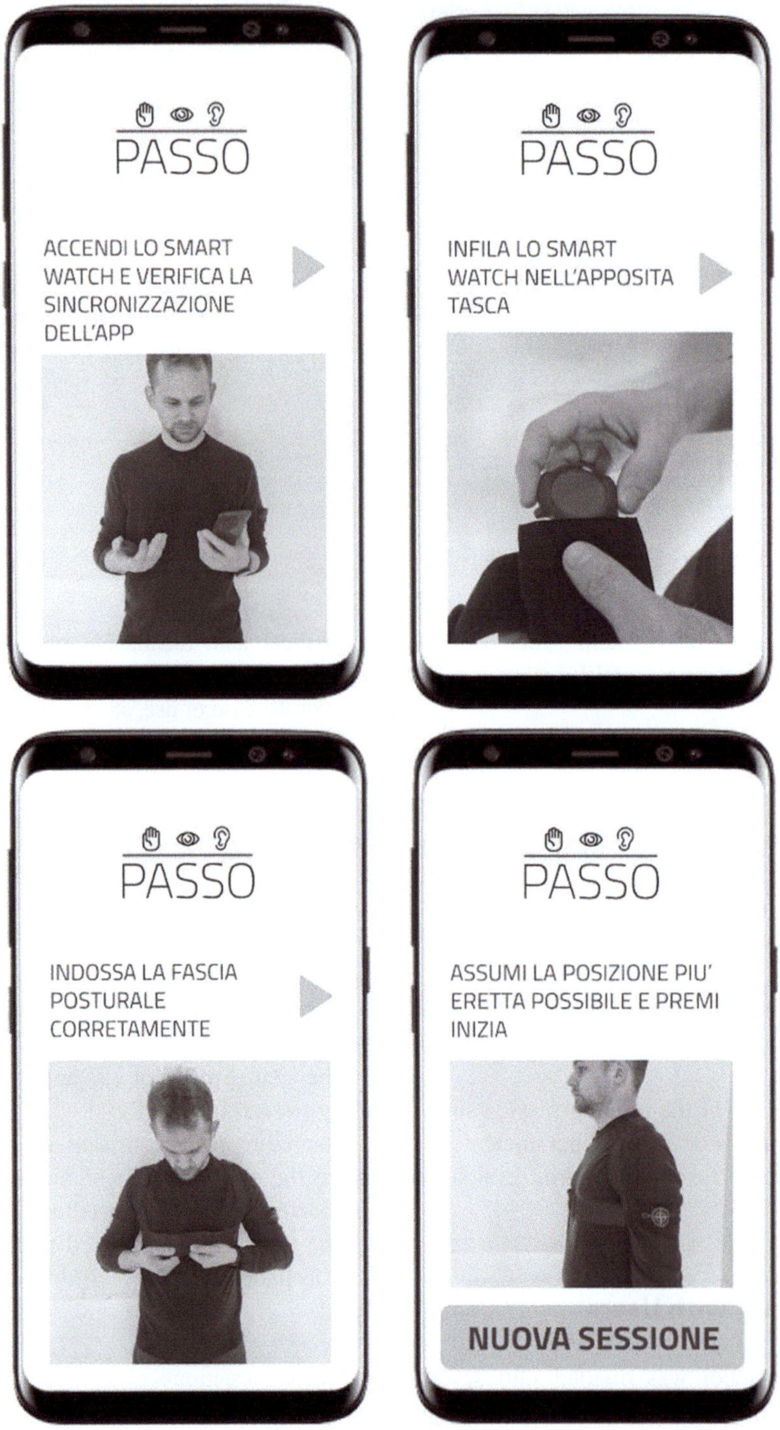

Fig. 9.7 Instruction to set the system and wear the Smart Harness before starting the training session

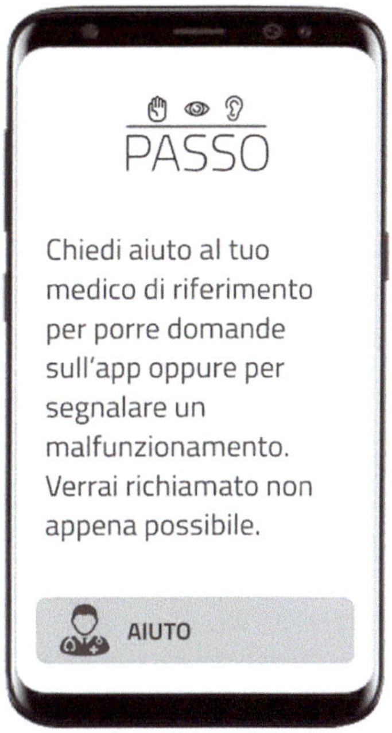

Fig. 9.8 Screen of the "Help" function

Hence, they were asked to carry out some tasks as Medical Operator:

- Access your profile
- Choose a specific patient profile from your list
- Create a new patient profile
- Change some parameters related to the patient
- Set parameters and thresholds for the patient's training session
- Look at a patient's past training sessions
- Start a new training session
- Look at the patient's new training session report

When it is possible to involve users with PD in the experimentation, they will be asked to practice the first part of the testing protocol, developed for their dedicated app version.

Testing Protocol for Medical and Technical Operators

Medical and Technical Operators testing the app were informally questioned about their impressions of the ease of use, accessibility, effectiveness, usability, and usefulness of the tested interfaces.

It was also elaborated a formal interview to be submitted to PD users when possible, asking about the user's perception of the system

Fig. 9.9 First screen for the Medical Operator where he can choose the patient who is going to be trained

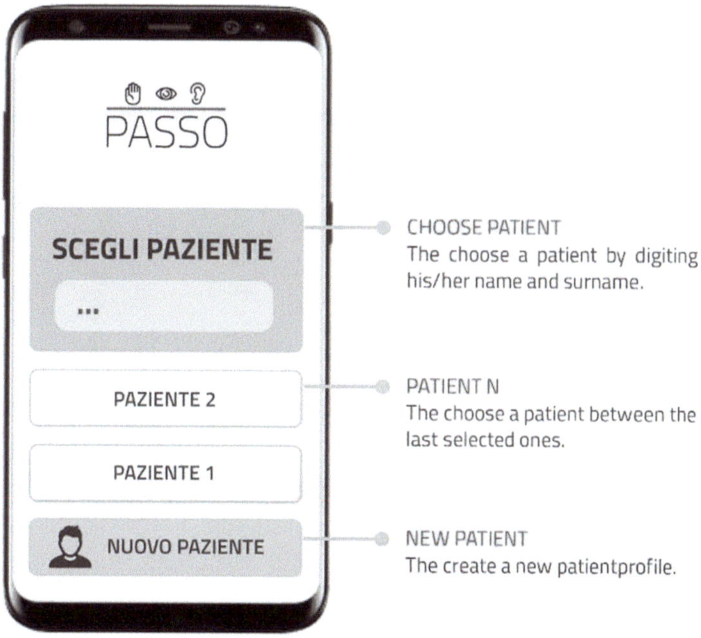

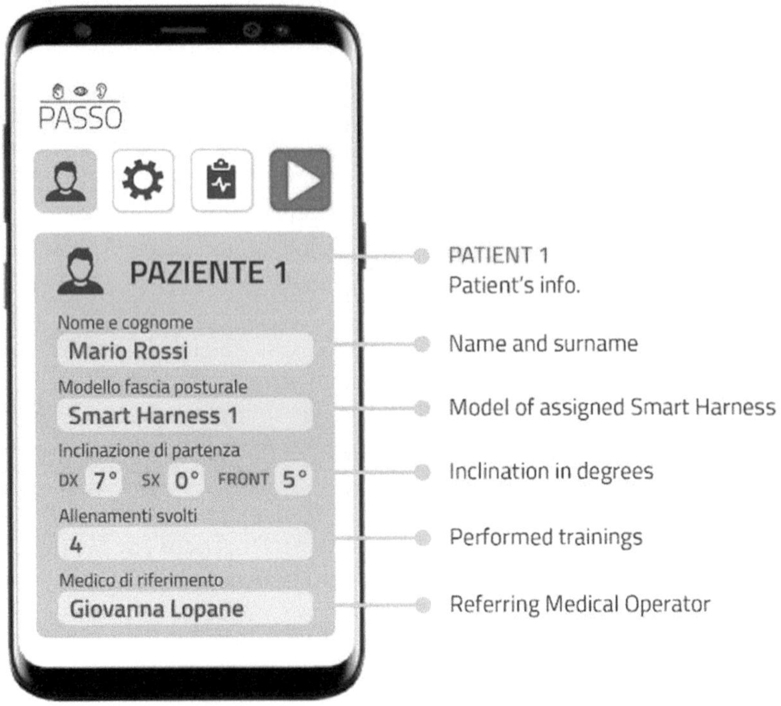

Fig. 9.10 Screen representing the patient profile

Fig. 9.11 Screen representing settings related to a specific patient

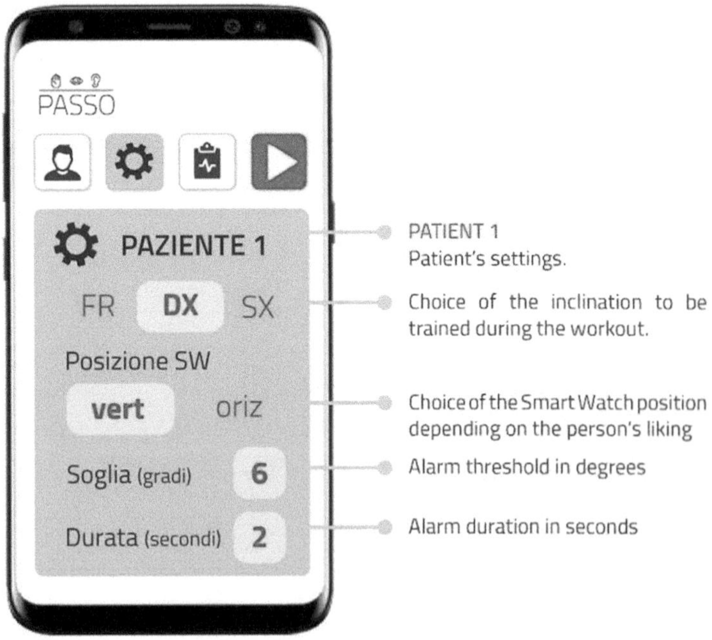

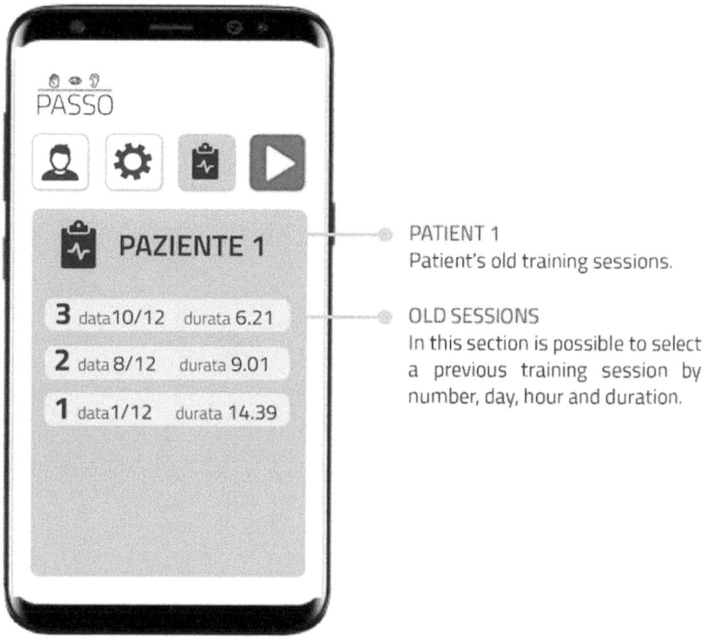

Fig. 9.12 Screen representing the person's previous training

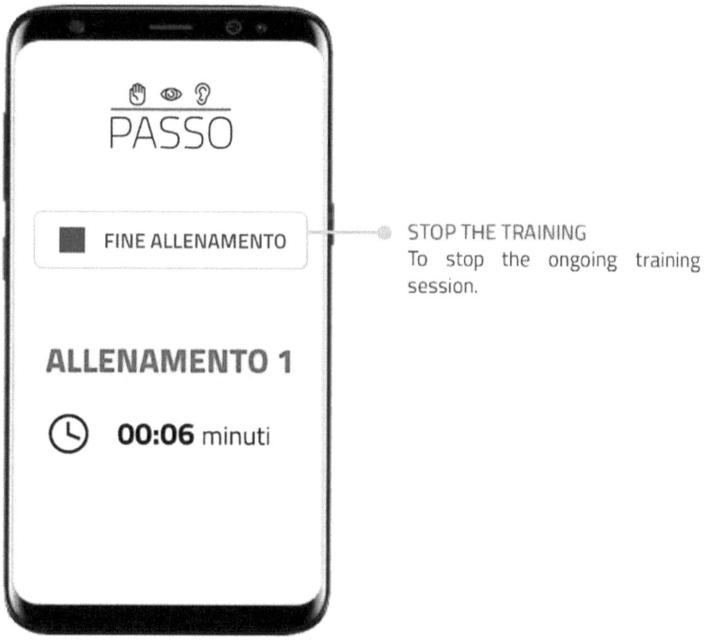

Fig. 9.13 Screen that the Medical Operator sees during the training session

interface, investigating his/her attitude to the system's functions, and discussing factors influencing perception.

During the first focus, the user will be free to comment on the screens as he prefers, without a structured list of questions. Secondly, he was asked/to give a mark from 1 to 5 to the needs reported in the following Table 9.1 (Tsai et al. 2020), giving the highest scores to the ones that he felt were his personal feelings. Needs listed in the table, grouped into different subcategories, will be collected to judge wearable smart

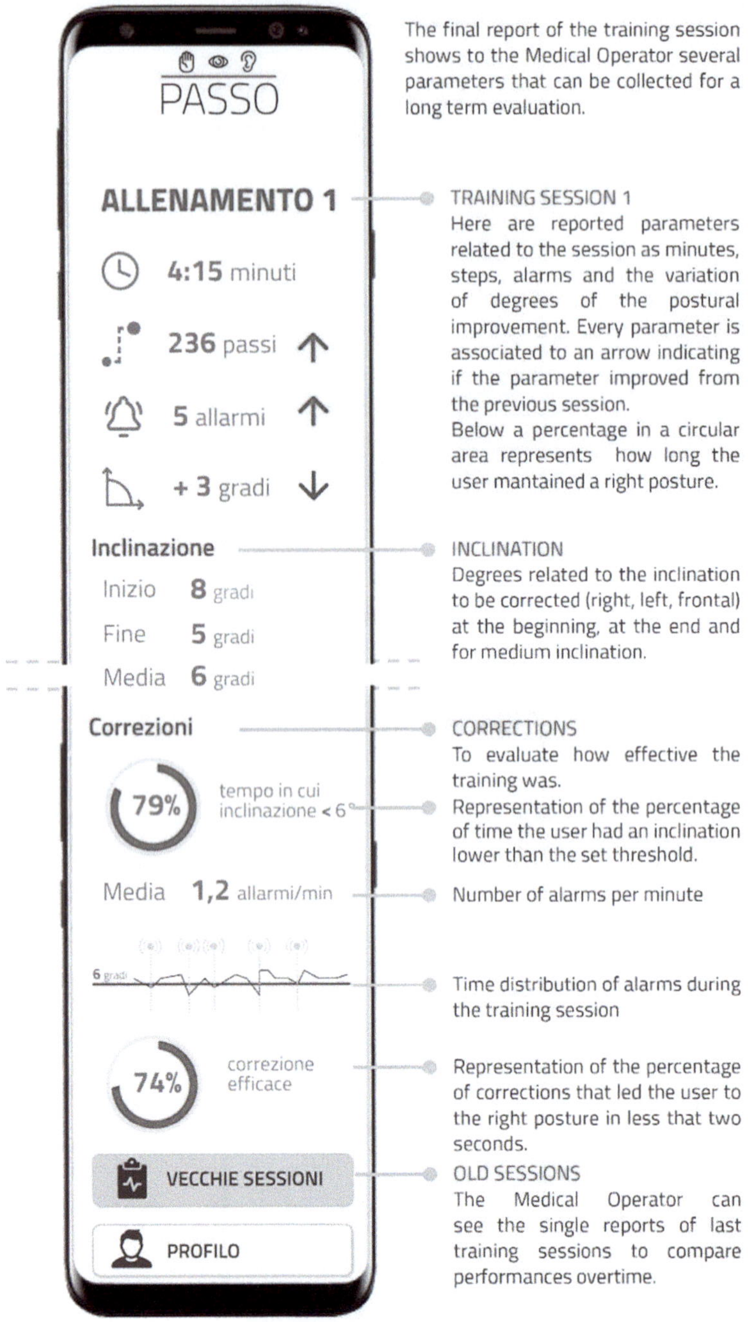

Fig. 9.14 Final report of the training session for the Medical Operator

Table 9.1 Table of characteristics importance

Variable	Description
Technology anxiety	I feel apprehensive about using the wearable system
	I hesitate to use technology for fear of making mistakes that I cannot correct
	I am afraid that the equipment may suddenly stop functioning
	I do not want other people to see me wearing smart devices
Perceived ubiquity	I want a wearable system that provides healthcare information "anytime and anywhere"
	The smart clothing system provides me with any-time and anywhere communication and connectivity
	I will use the smart clothing system very often for health purposes
Resistance to change	I do not want the smart clothing system to change the way I deal with related problems
	I do not want the smart system to change the way I keep myself healthy
	I do not want the smart system to change the way I interact with other people
	Overall, I do not want the smart system to change the way I currently live
Perceived usefulness	Using smart devices will improve my life quality
	Using the smart system will make my life more convenient
	Using the smart system will make me more effective in my life
	Overall, I find the smart system to be useful in my life
Perceived ease of use	I want the smart system to be clear and understandable
	I think that the smart clothing system does not require a lot of mental effort
	I find the smart clothing system to be easy to use
Attitude	I think that using the smart clothing system is a good idea
	I think that using the smart clothing system is beneficial to me
	I have a positive perception of using the smart clothing system
Behavioral intention	I intend to use the smart clothing system in the future
	I will always try to use the smart clothing system in my daily life
	I plan to use the smart clothing system frequently

systems giving a user vision of the developed solutions (Imbesi and Scataglini 2021).

9.3 Quantitative and Qualitative Evaluations

It is not possible to make complete evaluations about the ongoing testing process missing PD users' points of view, but it is possible to make some first considerations.

In Technical Operators' opinion, the interface conceived for users with PD takes a very low cognitive effort not bothering the user with long procedures for simple tasks. It contains only fundamental functions, not giving them the possibility to modify settings or to get lost in unknown parameters. Regarding the medical profile, Technical Operators appreciated the simplification of procedures and information and suggested adding in the app the possibility of interaction between Technical and Medical Operators.

Considering Medical Operators' opinions, the version for users with PD was simple and easy to use. Graphic solutions were appreciated for their accessibility and inclusivity, limiting the effort of required fine motor skills. Furthermore, the version dedicated to Medical Operators was described as simple and aesthetically pleasing, not creating a sense of being in a deeply technical environment. Specifically, the form used for the performance report was considered very effective and accessible in its reading and comprehension, avoiding complex graphics and parameters that are difficult to interpret by a medical professional.

9.4 Conclusions

At the moment it is possible to say that for both designed interfaces, one of the most appreciated aspects is a simplification.

Talking about the interface for users with PD, it was chosen to give the patient only information easy to understand at first sight. In this perspective, only fundamental functions were inserted using as few screens as possible and limiting gestures to "tap" and vertical "drag" to facilitate people with motor impairments. For the graphic aspect, a simple font designed for an on-screen display was chosen. The size of letters and the choice of strong contrasts in the color palette were aimed at helping those with visual and cognitive impairments. The design of buttons and layout wanted to give an intuitive interpretation of how to fulfill desired tasks.

Medical Operators were satisfied with the interface's intuitiveness, not making them feel overwhelmed by a large amount of information as often happens in technical settings conceived from the Technical Operators' perspective and not from the Medicals' one. Another element positively considered was the final report because of the easy interpretation and the friendly graphics. The color palette was the same as the other version, due to its saturation contrasts considered helpful in visualization. Also, the font choice was maintained but, otherwise, the dimensions of letters and buttons were reduced.

Medical Operators even appreciated the possibility of setting training parameters by themselves quickly and easily, needing less help from Technical Operators.

Personalization is confirmed to be a fundamental aspect of the satisfaction of users' needs.

At the moment, the interface in its two versions is a mockup of the app, and it does not interact with the system. This stage will be implemented after testing the current version with PD users and applying suggested improvements. Then, it will be possible to test a working version of the app, currently remotely activated by a Technical Operator.

Medical Operators suggested the possibility of having schemes representing performance trends over time. This was initially considered but not developed because it could be visually complex. They also suggested the possibility of integrating with the patient's profile some information external to the application but useful for comparisons given a long-term evaluation of the patient's performance.

When the final interface is designed, it will be installed on the smartphones of some doctors and patients of the Istituto delle Scienze Neurologiche di Bologna (ISBN), in the Bellaria Hospital of Bologna, Italy. Doctors will use the application in ambulatory contexts during medical examinations to set specific and personalized workouts for each patient. Patients will use the application when training themself on their own in indoor or outdoor environments, according to medical prescriptions, while wearing the Smart Harnessand. They will have to report regularly to the doctor their goals and frustrations to make the training effective.

Even in this design cycle, UCD led to satisfactory results, transforming the involvement of users into a useful design tool. The needs collection and the application of the QFD tool allowed the definition of characteristics most impacting on this design cycle, considered in the development of prototypes.

From the previous phases, it was evident that the interface should give users only fundamental information to avoid mistakes and uncomfortable feelings about using the app, which often are the primary reasons causing a loss of motivation to use it. For apps related to health management, it is important to maintain and, if possible, improve motivation. This can be done thanks to accessibility and usability. Moreover, even for people using an app for work reasons, it is fundamental to consider usability as an important objective.

Besides, usability and accessibility are both sustained by graphic choices that have a central role in facilitating intuitiveness and ease of use. The selection of specific fonts, shapes, dimensions, and color palettes guarantees the highest efficiency in completing tasks.

The development of an innovative interface in its simplicity, practicality, and application seems to be able to provide a positive and constructive stimulus in the constancy of use and long-term federalization.

References

S. Imbesi, S. Scataglini, A user centered methodology for the design of smart apparel for older users. Sensors **21**(8), 8 (2021). https://doi.org/10.3390/s21082804

J. Johnson, K. Finn, *Designing User Interfaces for an Aging Population: Towards Universal Design* (Morgan Kaufmann, 2017)

P. Maziewski, P. Suchomski, B. Kostek, A. Czyzewski, An intuitive graphical user interface for the Parkinson's Disease patients, in *2009 4th International IEEE/EMBS Conference on Neural Engineering* (2009), pp. 14–17. https://doi.org/10.1109/NER.2009.5109223

F. Nunes, P.A. Silva, J. Cevada, A. Correia Barros, L. Teixeira, User interface design guidelines for smartphone applications for people with Parkinson's disease. Univ. Access Inf. Soc. **15**(4), 659–679 (2016). https://doi.org/10.1007/s10209-015-0440-1

T.-H. Tsai, W.-Y. Lin, Y.-S. Chang, P.-C. Chang, M.-Y. Lee, Technology anxiety and resistance to change behavioral study of a wearable cardiac warming system using an extended TAM for older adults. PLoS ONE **15**(1), e0227270 (2020). https://doi.org/10.1371/journal.pone.0227270

K.L. Young, S. Koppel, J.L. Charlton, Toward best practice in Human Machine Interface design for older drivers: a review of current design guidelines. Accid. Anal. Prev. **106**, 460–467 (2017). https://doi.org/10.1016/j.aap.2016.06.010

Considerations on the Project 10

Abstract

The PASSO design research project was composed of three separated design cycles following a User-Centered approach: the first regarded the design of sensory cues rehabilitating the gait and posture of people with Parkinson's disease, the second was about the design of a smart wearable device submitting vibrating signals for rehabilitation training, and the last third one focused on the design of the web app managing the smart system functioning. This last chapter of the book has a particular structure that resumes the final considerations of each design cycle of the project and gives general conclusions about the adopted methodology and its potentialities in the application to other project addresses to niche fragile users.

10.1 General Conclusions About the PASSO Project

In this last chapter, the author resumes the conclusions of each single design cycle and the entire PASSO project. The obtained results are relevant, especially from the methodological point of view, because this research project allowed the possibility to design and validate a rigorous human-centered methodology conceived for complex innovative projects carried out by multidisciplinary research teams (Imbesi 2022).

This chapter's sections are structured as paragraphs each one reporting a consideration, expressed by a sentence at the beginning of the paragraph, about an interesting or innovative aspect of the design research project and its cycles (Imbesi and Corzani 2023; Imbesi and Mincolelli 2022; Imbesi et al. 2021).

In the current socioeconomic global scenario, it is strategic to invest in research for the elderly

It is well known that in the last decades the global population, especially in the most developed countries, is getting older. This scenario is significantly affecting public expenses related to older people's healthcare, giving a burden to younger generations. The current growth of elder people seems to be a solid trend that will not change in the short term, which is why it would be desirable to greatly improve welfare expenses in research for products, services, systems, and processes for healthcare purposes, especially for the prevention of age-related diseases. Promoting healthy aging, impairments prevention, and health parameters monitoring, can improve the quality of life not only for older users but for the whole society.

S. Imbesi, *Inclusive Design of a Smart Device for People with Parkinson's Disease*, Design For Inclusion 4, https://doi.org/10.1007/978-3-031-58249-3_10

Multidisciplinarity is indispensable in innovative research projects

Research fields mainly involved in the PASSO project were design, engineering, and medicine. The complexity of the whole project, articulated in many stages and necessitating a contribution by several scientific disciplines, was faced thanks to the composition of a multidisciplinary research group working towards design-driven innovation.

Design Research provides design methodologies to facilitate the design process involving different typologies of professionals, the applied one was the Quality Function Deployment tool. Moreover, a special focus was dedicated to the communication, explication, and representation of technical aspects and concepts to allow a deeper understanding of the ongoing results of the design process to every professional of the multidisciplinary research group. The visual representation of information like data, tables, and functions was inclusive and accessible improving the involvement of researchers in the project.

UCD applied to digital technologies as an up-and-coming area of research

At the intersection between UC design methods and digital technologies, there is an up-and-coming area of research, which will have to produce many fruits relatively quickly to mitigate the impact of global aging and offer new sustainable solutions to support active and healthy aging. This research faces a timely and significant challenge related to the global aging of the population and the subsequent burden of age-related diseases and syndromes, proposing an innovative methodological solution.

Methodological guidelines for multidisciplinary UC Design Research

The main prospective impact of this doctoral research is supposed to be in the advancement of methodological guidelines for the design of UC solutions for older people affected by PD. This area is particularly challenging due to the need to integrate multi-disciplinary teams and a heterogeneous body of knowledge.

However, when validated on a larger sample, the proposed methodology might pave the way for a new generation of smart devices.

Research project as a set of interrelated but projectually independent stages

The field of mobility aids for mitigating the consequences of PD-related movement disorders seems to deserve further R&D contributions. This research explored design methodologies that could become a reference in the sector.

The choice of an iterative User-Centered Design methodology divided into three iterative cycles (organized in four phases and linked with achieving a specific TRL) is interesting in this field because it offers the possibility of splitting up the project into several stages that can be addressed separately, and each one can give rise to different and parallel lines of innovative research.

Encountered issues related to coronavirus as momentaneus limitations for the project

The Coronavirus pandemic suddenly brought unexpected issues and delays to the doctoral research planned activities. It was necessary to change some aspects of the ongoing research to manage the situation and plan a new strategy. The most significant problem was the impossibility for a long period to physically involving older PD users in the trial due to the risk of contagion. Even difficulties with team meetings in person momentarily dulled the enthusiasm of the researchers. All issues were solved thanks to the extra time given for the research completion.

Experimental results achieved involving and testing different categories of users (healthy subjects, clinicians, and patients), gave clear results but the ongoing experimentation, involving a supplementary sample of people with PD, will contribute to the project validation.

The obtained results are coherent with dedicated scientific literature.

10.2 Considerations on the Project Cycles

Design project as the composition of UCD cycles

The three UCD cycles composing the project gave each one its results, they can be considered separately and all together to make punctual or general considerations from the methodological and technical points of view.

Every design cycle followed the same scheme composed of four design phases: Planning, Analyzing, Creating, and Verifying.

Division of the project into cycles with their objectives and strategies led to multiple objectives and conclusions

The adopted methodology consented to developing each design cycle as a sort of independent project, strongly correlated with the others, allowing the definition of punctual objectives and different design strategies. The choice of the consequentiality of the cycles was determined by how the results of one would be the starting points for the next. At the end of the project, it is possible to say that each project cycle brought results that, even if considered separately from the results of the other cycles, can be considered an innovative contribution to the field of research that combines UCD and advanced digital health technologies addressed to older users affected by PD.

Considerations on Cycle 1

Sensory cues were experimented with using earphones and Smart Glasses. Auditory cues were the ones obtaining the most effective results in influencing the gait, especially the ones using traditional musical instruments. Vibratory cues gave promising results, especially in light of the limitations given by the device. Results suggested that visual cues are not strategic for temporal signals as cadence. Nevertheless, all the cues improved users' gait

In cycle 1 were tested auditory cues by earphones and visual and vibratory cues by SG.

As shown in the developed process, auditory cues were the most effective ones, then we had the vibratory ones followed by the multisensory, and at last, there were visual cues.

Interestingly, among the winning cues for the auditory channel, the classic metronome (B1) achieved 9%, the lowest percentage. Besides, with 11% the winner is the melody composed of musical instruments and electronic sounds (B3). Compared to the classic metronome, the users perceive it as less annoying, and they can reach the target cadence imposed by the rhythm with fewer steps. Differently, signals with traditional musical instruments were considered less bothersome and more calming because of their similarity to natural human sounds.

Vibratory cues were a little less performing than the auditory ones; it is possible to compare them to the metronome. On the other hand, the possibility of transmitting this signal only by the SG lenses seemed to limit significantly the potential of feedback using this sensory channel.

Visual cues received the worst scores, and the possible reason could be that this typology of cues is appropriate for training related to space perception, but is not suitable for the submission of temporal information to be followed, as the cadence.

Nevertheless, compared to the baseline trial, all the cues tested appear to induce a more symmetrical gait and a reduction in gait variability, confirming the positive role of the cueing strategy.

The closer the imposed stimuli's rhythm is to the person's cadence, the more the cue is effective. Visual cueing affects primarily spatial gait parameters while auditory and somatosensory cueing primarily improve temporal gait features. Unimodal feedback for the user is less overwhelming than the multimodal ones.

Interestingly, from radar plot analysis, it is clear that the imposed stimuli's rhythm (fixed at 100 [step/min]) is slightly lower than that of the subjects. This led to a reduction in their stride length and gait speed, as well as an increase in their cadence variability as a consequence of the newly imposed rhythm.

It is known that different cueing modalities have a differential effect on gait rehabilitation: during the verifying phase it was confirmed that while visual cueing primarily improves spatial gait parameters (e.g., stride length), auditory and somatosensory cueing primarily improves temporal gait features (e.g., gait speed and cadence). QFD outcomes align with these indications: all the auditory and vibratory feedback reach a higher percentage than the visual ones.

In addition, obtained outcomes indicated that the unimodal feedback is more effective than the multimodal one which in some cases was perceived as bothersome and confusing. The aspect of unimodal cues' prowess could be partially linked to the choice of a simple walking paradigm, in which the subject had to walk on a linear path without obstruction, trying to adapt to the suggested cadence rhythm.

The system's overall functioning, its tested usability, and effectiveness demonstrated by most of the cues, made it possible to assess the achievement of TRL 5, thanks to the laboratory testing protocols.

Critical points detected in this cycle were the synchronization between gait and signal beginning, the difference between suggested and user's cadence, and the user's sense preferences influencing their perception.

From this first design cycle, according to detected parameters, it was possible to identify critical points such as the synchronization between the submission of the signal and the person's gait phase, the discrepancy between the person's cadence and the one suggested by the system, and the haptic cue's location confined to the single SG's temples.

Another limitation of the described approach was the extent to which each subject is visual-, auditory-, or somatosensory-dependent: the nervous system uses augmented sensory information differently depending primarily on individual proclivities to rely on one sensory channel over another to control motor behavior.

To overcome some of these limitations, the target cadence should be subject-specific and based on the one detected during a user's reference gait during gait training. Alternatively, the target cadence could be an edited version of the one registered during the user's reference walk.

UCD methodologies allow for the reduction of complexity in multidisciplinary design processes. this design cycle could continue as an autonomous line of research.

Considering the methodological strategy, the results of this first UCD design cycle are satisfactory and encouraging for the next phases. Besides, the experimented UCD methodology, especially the verifying phase (C1P4), has proven to reduce the complexity of multidisciplinary design processes involving human and technological aspects challenging to compare.

This cycle can be evaluated as an own standing project. In this case, its individual future development could be related to new protocols verifying demanding paths instead of a linear walk, using visual cues to advise about spatial obstacles in the environment rather than to suggest a cadence, related to temporal parameters.

Considerations on Cycle 2

During the second cycle, vibratory cues were tested developing an innovative wearable device using a smartwatch for the correction of posture.

From the previous cycle, it was decided to develop vibratory cues, in the light of their potential, but transmitted with the correct device. During the first cycle, the best results were given by auditory cues influencing the gait, in this cycle it was decided to study deep vibratory cues for the correction of posture. Thanks to scientific literature and some informal experiments involving the multidisciplinary team, it was decided to focus on vibrations transmitted on the person's trunk.

The second design cycle aimed to design and test a system based on vibratory cues, using a new tailored wearable device. It was decided to experiment with the combined use of SWs with a postural band, obtaining a smart harness, and submitting haptic cues to influence the person's posture. Specifically, the smart wearable device was conceived to correct frontal and mediolateral inclination.

The most effective signals are the ones using a smartwatch at a time. Customization in vibration modality and positioning and the wearable device model and size improved usability. The system allows a posture evaluation in real time and transmits haptic cues to correct inclination. The testing protocol showed corrections were evident and appreciable.

After testing different configurations, it was observed that the best cues for clarity and ease of interpretation were the ones involving only a single SW at a time. This choice was fundamentally linked to the clinician's goal: for a patient with PD, it is important to define one and only one clinical target to improve his most impaired function. The simultaneous attempt to correct more than one gait or posture aspect at the same time could induce the PD person to cognitive overload, making him feel overwhelmed; on the contrary, the request of a single task allows the patient to focus only on that goal, making his performance more effective (for example, for subjects with Pisa Syndrome, it is enough one SW on the compromised lateral side that acts as a reminder every time needed). Acting like this, the developed mHealth system allows high customization and could be used for specific clinical needs.

Personalization is fundamental in smart devices addressed to PD users. Used smart harnesses were adjustable in size, increasing the fit and wearability of the wearable device, but they were also perceived differently by users, depending on their body (for example, women chose the second model of the smart harness because it did not press their chest). Even the positioning of the SW in the smart harness was not felt in the same way by patients, (for example, in the case of frontal inclination most of the users preferred to have the SW positioned on the chest, but some others felt uncomfortable with this configuration and preferred the model positioning the SW on their back between the shoulder blades).

Moreover, considering the system, its logging capability allowed the possibility of an overall evaluation of the postural performance immediately after the session or after a certain number of training sessions. Parameters about the user's postural behavior with cues are stored within the device and can be automatically monitored over several days.

Users involved in the project participated in a testing protocol to monitor their posture in a linear path without any signal, in a linear path with the submission of haptic cues, and finally in a path with everyday obstacles with the submission of haptic cues. Technical Operators analyzed the micro and macro outcomes from the trunk angle information to describe the specific tests performed. The obtained parameters confirmed the potential of the device to improve the person's posture.

UCD helped in managing and organizing the design process and involving users in each stage of the design process improving the response to their needs. QFD suggested characteristics on which to focus more and unsatisfied users' needs.

Even in this second cycle, UCD proved to be an effective tool for managing and organizing the design process. Experiments carried out with the help of primary and secondary users led to satisfactory solutions from a qualitative point of view, testifying a high degree of wearability, usability, and accessibility of the whole system.

The whole multidisciplinary team was involved in the elaboration of the QFD matrix, thanks to graphical strategies everybody could understand considerations made by members belonging to a different research field. The QFD tool gave as output a list of importance of measurable characteristics belonging to the developed device and system. Results obtained till now confirm the hierarchization of characteristics expressed by results of the QFD.

Prototypes of harnesses and systems were tested by users to confirm aspects related to ergonomics and usability.

This cycle could continue as an autonomous project making it also a tele-rehabilitation system.

Imagining this design cycle as a single project, it would be very interesting to continue the testing phase giving the users the smart devices and letting them have training sessions in their environments by themselves, using the project also as a tele-rehabilitation smart device. A potential advantage of this solution would be the possible continuous training for an extended period in a real-life scenario, a key element in the rehabilitation of chronic diseases, such as PD. Besides, the postural trunk features computed by the system may also be exploited in the future as methods to assess postural control, both in a clinical context and more interestingly in an out-of-the-lab environment.

Considerations on Cycle 3

During the last design cycle, an app for the system interface was developed and tested. The version dedicated to users with PD was appreciated for its simplification of graphics, gestures, and functions. The version for Medical Operators was described as intuitive, complete in functions, and graphically pleasing. Personalization is confirmed to be a relevant aspect.

The third and last design cycle of the PASSO project aimed to design a smartphone application for the mHealth system management in two versions, one developed for the personal training of the person with PD, and the other one created for Medical Operators practicing this kind of rehabilitation program.

The design of the user interfaces has taken into consideration graphic solutions aimed at guaranteeing maximum accessibility to all users, even those with specific cognitive and motor needs. Considering that users with PD have not yet been involved in all the testing phases, it is now possible to consider only the Operator's point of view for the evaluation of the app's patient version.

For both designed interfaces, one of the most appreciated aspects was simplification. The interface for users with PD was chosen to give the patient only information easy to understand at first sight. In this perspective, only fundamental functions were inserted using as few screens as possible and limiting gestures to "tap" and vertical "drag" to facilitate people with motor impairments. For the graphic aspect, a simple font designed for an on-screen display was chosen. The size of letters and the choice of strong contrasts in the color palette were aimed at helping those with visual and cognitive impairments. The design of buttons and layout wanted to give an intuitive interpretation of how to fulfill desired tasks.

Medical Operators were satisfied with the interface's intuition, not making them feel overwhelmed by a large amount of information as often happens in technical settings conceived from the Technical Operators' perspective and not from the medical one. Another element positively considered was the final report because of the easy interpretation and the friendly graphics. The color palette was the same as the other version, due to its saturation contrasts considered helpful in visualization. Also, the font choice was maintained but, otherwise, the dimensions of letters and buttons were reduced.

Medical Operators even appreciated the possibility of setting training parameters by themselves quickly and easily, needing less help from Technical Operators.

Personalization is confirmed to be a fundamental aspect of the satisfaction of users' needs.

Medical Operators suggested the possibility of having schemes representing performance trends over time. This was initially considered but not developed because it could be visually complex. They also suggested the possibility of integrating into the patient's profile some information external to the application but useful for comparisons given a long-term evaluation of the patient's performance.

UCD was useful in involving users in the definition of the project's requirements and its validation. Graphics have a fundamental role in guaranteeing the interface's usability and accessibility.

Even in this design cycle, UCD led to satisfactory results, transforming the involvement of users into a useful design tool. The needs collection and the application of the QFD tool allowed the definition of characteristics most impacting on this design cycle, considered in the development of prototypes.

From the previous phases, it emerged that the interface should give users only fundamental information to avoid mistakes and uncomfortable feelings about using the app, which often are the primary reasons causing a loss of motivation to use it. For apps related to health management, it is important to maintain and, if possible, improve motivation. This can be done thanks to accessibility and usability. Moreover, even for people using an app for work reasons, it is fundamental to consider usability as an important objective.

Besides, usability and accessibility are both sustained by graphic choices that have a central role in facilitating intuitiveness and ease of use. The selection of specific fonts, shapes, dimensions, and color palettes guarantees the highest efficiency in completing tasks.

The development of an innovative interface in its simplicity, practicality, and application seems to be able to provide a positive and constructive stimulus in the constancy of use and long-term federalization.

In future developments, the system will be used by patients in their environments.

The current app version will be implemented in a beta-testing system. When the final interface is completed, it will be installed on the smartphones of some doctors and patients of the Istituto delle Scienze Neurologiche di Bologna (ISBN), in the Bellaria Hospital of Bologna, Italy. Doctors will use the application in ambulatory contexts during medical examinations to set specific and personalized workouts for each patient. Patients will use the application when training themself on their own in indoor or outdoor environments, according to medical prescriptions, while wearing the Smart Harness. They will have to report regularly to the doctor their goals and frustrations to make the training effective.

References

S. Imbesi, Human-centered design for older users: a design methodology for the development of smart devices and systems related to health Care, in *Internet of Things for Human-Centered Design: Application to Elderly Healthcare. Studies in Computational Intelligence*, ed. by S. Scataglini, S. Imbesi, G. Marques (Springer Nature, Singapore, 2022), pp. 25–37. https://doi.org/10.1007/978-981-16-8488-3_2

S. Imbesi, M. Corzani, Multisensory cues for gait rehabilitation with smart glasses: methodology, design, and results of a preliminary pilot. Sensors **23**(2) (2023). https://doi.org/10.3390/s23020874

S. Imbesi, G. Mincolelli, Design of a rehabilitation system monitoring gait of users with Parkinson's disease: data visualization as a methodological tool, in *Digital Human Modeling and Applied Optimization* (AHFE Open Access, 2022). https://doi.org/10.54941/ahfe1001907

S. Imbesi, M. Corzani, F. Petrocchi, G. Lopane, L. Chiari, G. Mincolelli, User-centered design of cues with smart glasses for gait rehabilitation in people with Parkinson's disease: a methodology for the analysis of human requirements and cues effectiveness, in *Advances in Simulation and Digital Human Modeling. Lecture Notes in Networks and Systems*, ed. by J.L. Wright, D. Barber, S. Scataglini, S.L. Rajulu (Springer International Publishing, Cham, 2021), pp. 348–358. https://doi.org/10.1007/978-3-030-79763-8_42

MIX
Papier aus verantwortungsvollen Quellen
Paper from responsible sources
FSC® C105338

If you have any concerns about our products,
you can contact us on
ProductSafety@springernature.com

In case Publisher is established outside the EU,
the EU authorized representative is:
Springer Nature Customer Service Center GmbH
Europaplatz 3, 69115 Heidelberg, Germany

Printed by Libri Plureos GmbH
in Hamburg, Germany